VISION
AND
HIGHWAY SAFETY

VISION
AND
HIGHWAY SAFETY

MERRILL J. ALLEN, O.D., PH.D.

PROFESSOR OF OPTOMETRY
INDIANA UNIVERSITY
BLOOMINGTON, INDIANA

PRINCIPLES OF <O>PTOMETRY SERIES
VOLUME ELEVEN

CHILTON BOOK COMPANY
PHILADELPHIA   NEW YORK   LONDON

Foreword

THIS BOOK is intended to provide optometrists, highway engineers, manufacturers, legislators, law enforcement personnel, and others with information on the visual aspects of driving a car. The optometrist will find information of value for the eye examination, for prescription of driving glasses, and for better understanding of the vision requirements for the driving task, all of which will be doubly helpful should he be called upon to serve as an expert witness in a court of law or to help shape legislation to improve highway safety.

Great efforts are now being made to improve the highway, the motor vehicle, and the training of the driver. Careful vision testing and elevated vision standards will ensure that the driver is fully prepared visually. And now that concerted efforts are being undertaken to improve the visual driving environment, both vehicular and highway, the driver will have the best possible visual surroundings.

It is hoped that this book will provide some of the information needed to help upgrade virtually all visual aspects of the driving task. The student interested in pursuing the details of the massive literature that is now available on the visual aspects of driving will find assistance in the bibliography.

Preface

PROFESSOR MERRILL ALLEN has been in the forefront of technical and policy concern over the visual environment provided by the contemporary automobile. His findings in the past have stimulated legislative and administrative action. In this book, he brings together his research and analysis as a direct challenge to the automobile industry to start reducing the strains on the driving task by removing known obstacles to driving vision and assisting the driver in coping with an ever more demanding highway environment. He also informs drivers of the myths and commercial banalities that impair and hinder their visual perception.

RALPH NADER

Contents

VISION
AND
HIGHWAY SAFETY

Chapter 1: Introduction

QUOTING automobile accident statistics is a popular approach to automotive safety. To be in step with the times, I will quote a few myself. That they are outdated, even as I write them, is a foregone conclusion. However, they will serve to indicate the magnitude of the problem and, I hope, give a different slant to the statistics usually presented.

It is reported that in 1899 the first automobile accident death was Henry H. Bliss, struck by an automobile in New York City. From 1900 to 1964 motor vehicle deaths in the United States totaled 1,510,000, while military deaths totaled only 605,000 from 1775 to 1964. (American Trial Lawyers' Association, 1966). Carrying the comparison farther, one notes that deaths among battle casualties in World War I were 8 percent of those reaching the hospital or medical installation. In World War II these deaths dropped to 4.5 percent, in the Korean War they were 2.5 percent, and in Vietnam they are about 2 percent. Of automobile deaths, 33 percent die at the scene, in the ambulance, or within minutes of arriving at the hospital (NAS, June 1969). Once the crash victim safely reaches the civilian hospital his chances of survival, it is hoped, are as good as they would be in Vietnam.

The number of drivers in 1967 was 103 million, of whom 13.5 million were involved in accidents. The number whose injuries caused at least a day of restricted activity or medical care was 3,535,000, or nearly 10,000 per day (DOT, 1969). Forty percent of all fatal accidents involve two or more motor vehicles. One out of three cars will cause an injury or death, and three out of four cars will be in an accident. In 1968 injuries, deaths, and property damage cost over 14.24 billion dollars and 55,500 deaths. Fantastic as these figures are, they still do not tell the sad story of the wounded veterans of the highway. Disfigurement and losses of bodily and mental function are the hidden costs. Many victims are permanently confined to a wheelchair or bed.

Statistics on visual disability caused by automobile accidents are hard to obtain, although all of us have seen patients with large phorias, diplopia, limited motility, facial scarring, and blindness resulting from

1

automobile injuries. Because the head is involved in about 75 percent of all injuries, the eyes, the orbit, and the supporting facial tissues come in for a large share of the trauma. The Cornell Aeronautical Laboratory reported in 1963 that 9.8 percent of the occupants injured in automobile accidents had ocular-orbital involvement. Of these, 92 percent suffered bruises, contusions, and minor and severe lacerations; only 4.2 percent had injuries to the eye itself, which attests to the remarkable protection offered by the orbit and to the "toughness" of the eye. If we apply Cornell's figure (Allen, 1964), and if we conservatively assume that the injury figure is 3,000,000, the number of people with ocular or orbital injuries is 294,000 per year. This is sufficient justification for optometrists to take a positive approach by encouraging their patients to use seat belts and shoulder harnesses.

With the annual increase in the number of cars and pedestrians, one can expect a continuing increase in the number of "accidents." It is hoped that deaths and injuries will begin to decline as the new safety features, first required by the General Services Administration and now by the National Traffic Safety Bureau of the Department of Transportation, are incorporated into new car production and as older cars are retired from the highways.

To what extent is vision involved in these accidents and to what extent is the visual status of the driver responsible for them? Analyses of accidents to determine the role played by measurable aspects of vision, such as visual acuity, color vision, and dark adaptation, have been disappointing. The most reliable studies to date are those from the Institute of Transportation and Traffic Engineering of the Department of Engineering of the University of California, Los Angeles, in cooperation with the California Department of Motor Vehicles. Starting in 1962, 17,500 test subjects were studied in depth. Summarizing these studies Burg, 1967, reports:

> "Among the vision variables studied, dynamic visual acuity shows the strongest and most consistent relationships with driving record. There is substantial but not conclusive evidence that static visual acuity, glare recovery, and visual field also are related to driving record.
> "The data suggest differential vision-driving relationships as a function of age; however, at the present stage of analysis, the precise nature and extent of these differential relationships cannot be determined.
> "The data strongly suggest differential vision-driving relationships as a function of sex. More definitive information will be provided by planned analyses involving specific accident types and qualitative exposure."

As to predicting a person's driving record, Burg, in the same report, states:

> "Among vision variables, the results support the original research hypothesis by showing that dynamic visual acuity is by far the most consistent contributor to prediction, followed by static acuity, glare recovery, and visual

field. The two remaining vision variables (glarimeter threshold and phoria) do not contribute consistently to prediction of a driving record variable; this does not imply that they might not contribute significantly in prediction of specific accident types, a possibility that future analyses will examine."

That alcohol is responsible for over 50 percent of the fatal accidents (Haddon et al., 1964); that mechanical failures contribute significantly to accident causation (Moseley et al., 1961–62 and 1962–63); that a significant number of "accidents" are murders, suicides, or both (Ford and Moseley, 1963); that a significant number are true accidents with no one at fault; that there is a high percentage of innocent victim involvement; and that there are many factors beside vision that determine driving success make Burg's accomplishment of relating vision to accidents all the more remarkable.

Other hazards to safe driving, such as carbon monoxide, tranquilizers, and antihistamines, act in part to destroy visual acuteness, visual motor coordination, and perceptual alertness. Any compensatable visual anomaly becomes progressively less compensatable under the influence of these agents. Darkness alone, for example, reduces the ability to fuse, to accommodate, and, for squinters, to suppress. In addition, the reaction time is increased, space judgments are altered, and alertness is reduced. One could expect that heavy smokers, all of whom show measurably higher levels of carbon monoxide in their blood (McFarland and Moseley, 1954), would have more asthenopia and more binocular vision and accommodative problems than persons not exposed to carbon monoxide; and that carbon monoxide symptoms would be increased at higher elevations above sea level (McFarland et al., 1944). The harmful effects of carbon monoxide on driving are at least aggravated by alcohol, darkness, and fatigue.

The magnitude of the visual problems in the population in America has been indicated in several studies. For example, it is reported that glaucoma exists in 2 percent of all over the age of forty; strabismus exists in from 2 to 7 percent of the population, while more than 8 percent have some form of color vision anomaly, about 17 percent have anisocoria to an extent which may be hazardous, and 0.5 to 4 percent have amblyopia; at grade school levels, 20 percent have visual anomalies sufficient to merit correction; and everyone by the age of sixty needs visual correction of some type.

A study of the population visiting the State Fair in Indiana (Allen, 1964) showed that visual deterioration with age was extensive. Field defects, ophthalmoscopic evidences of pathology, and visual inadequacy at far and/or near went up with age, particularly among women over forty years old. Most people tested were capable of normal vision but had not taken steps to obtain it. Probably these statistics were colored by self-selection. People in poor health may have come to the test booth in higher numbers than those who believed their vision was corrected.

In the interests of retaining driving privileges, almost everyone would seek vision care. To identify people with problems like those seen at the State Fair, the quality of motor vehicle department vision testing and test standards for driver licensure must be improved. Knowledgeable optometrists should cooperate with and monitor the license bureau testing stations to ensure effective visual screening. The conservative attitude of professionals who fear that their efforts will be construed as a bid to get more patients is no longer a valid excuse. When the men who know the problems and the needs fail to speak out, the public suffers through reduced efficiency, increased fatigue, more injuries, and more deaths.

Continuing to permit drivers with substandard vision to operate a vehicle because it is difficult to prove the need for superior vision draws a parallel with practices in the automobile industry and elsewhere that are based upon economics, expediency, or styling, and not vision. Automobile manufacturers and others for nearly fifty years refused to incorporate safety features until safety advocates proved that what was proposed would save lives. It is now finally becoming possible for outsiders to reverse the position and to ask the manufacturers to prove the superiority of such things as, for example, windshield design, signal systems, or dash panel design. Vision experts must no longer be tricked into tolerating less than optimum vision design features of the products offered for sale simply because of expediency in manufacture, the influence of marketing factors unrelated to visual efficiency, and the fact that next year's car has already been designed and "cannot be changed." When the manufacturer asks for proof that the visually correct way is better, he should be asked in turn to show justification for the hazardous or nonoptimum approach he has used. This applies not only to automobiles but also to bathroom mirror illumination, desk lamps, lawn mowers, window glass, and, yes, even spectacle frames and lenses.

The idea that the need for a pair of glasses might cause an accident is a simplification of the visual factors entering into safe driving. Certainly, without vision there can be no driving of today's automobiles. No other sense modality holds such a veto power. Yet good vision alone is not enough to drive a motor vehicle. It is the myriad of other factors that makes the job of the scientist so difficult when he tries to prove the degree to which vision affects driving! This book will give the reader a greater appreciation of the complexities of the problem as well as some recommendations about what can be done to reduce accidents.

Chapter 2: The Driving Task

WHAT is the nature of the problem facing the driver? What does he have to do and what information is available to him? Aside from the simplicity of the statement that the driving task is the task of operating a motor vehicle from point A to point B without an accident, the computer approach is more satisfying.

Figure 2-1 provides a diagrammatic representation of a major portion of the driving task. The eye is the only source of driver information about objects on the roadway; that is, their speed, size, course, and possibly hazardous nature. It is the only source of information on roadway signs, traffic signals, and vehicle signals. In addition it is the most important feedback source of information on the effect of compensatory or other motor action of the driver. Such actions as steering, braking, or accelerating also supply information to the brain via the ears, vestibular apparatus, and pressure sensors at various other points in the body.

If a system involving a roadway, a driver, and a vehicle is to work properly, the driver must have proper knowledge, memory, and experience; a reliable and predictably responsive machine; and a proportional feedback from the environment by way of his several sense modalities.

That these ideal conditions do not usually exist in the present-day driving situation is little appreciated by most people. There are numerous and serious sources of interference (or noise) in the information supplied to the driver. Let us take an easily understood mechanical system, such as power brakes, and evaluate the feedback to the driver. First the driver presses his foot on the brake pedal. For a distance of one half to two inches of pedal travel no braking effect occurs, and the pedal force is perhaps one and a half pounds. Then a travel of about one half inch more at a pedal force of often no more than about three pounds is enough to lock all four wheels. This alone can be very disturbing to a driver. Now consider what happens when braking commences. The tires gripping the road pull back on the axles, which, through assorted linkages and rubber vibration dampers, transmit the force to the frame. At a measurable length of time after the brakes are applied, the automobile body starts to slow down. The driver begins to slow down when the

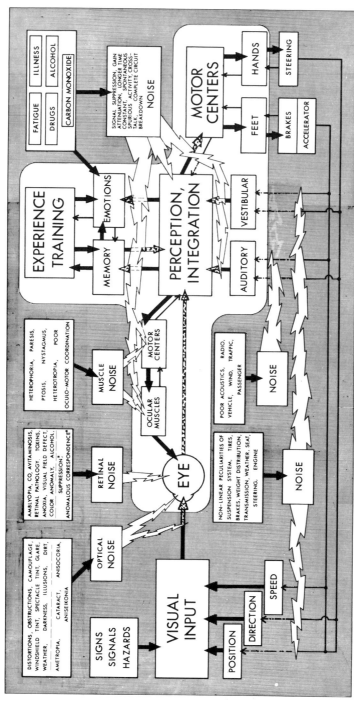

Figure 2-1. A schematic diagram of the driving task. The visual input into the eye is the beginning of a closed loop which proceeds via the perception-integration and motor control centers of the brain through the hands and feet, the vehicle, the position on the road, and finally back to the visual input. The lightning streaks represent potential or real interferences which operate to reduce the effi-ciency of the driver. The main arrows show interference (noise) by being drawn as spotty. Note that the brain is able to sort out the noise and obtain surprisingly accurate information. Because of the brain's ability, few realize how much impairment occurs in every-day driving that may become serious if the brain's ability is com-promised by fatigue, illness, lack of training, or overloading.

springs and the sponge rubber padding in the seat have been put under tension by the slowing of the car. In other words, he tends to slide forward toward the instrument panel. This forward movement of his body when his foot is on the brake increases the braking action as a positive feedback mechanical interaction. The increased brake action causes him to slide forward still more, putting on still more brake. To avoid locking wheels, the driver must attempt to lift his foot off the brake pedal just enough to control wheel lock and yet to obtain maximum brake effect, allowing of course for the time delay when the positive feedback commences. Great coordination and much practice are necessary to make a smooth stop by releasing brake pressure just enough to compensate for positive feedback. This is an almost impossible feat in a crisis.

There is little doubt that this positive feedback mechanical coupling is responsible for loss of vehicle control and rear-end accidents or skids on wet or icy streets. That accidents may have been averted by having such sensitive brakes is possible, but the loss of vehicle control and the reduction of braking efficiency resulting when wheels lock must be viewed in their true light as accident-producing characteristics.

Let us take a look on the other hand at a smoothly operating self-limiting (negative feedback) control system, the automobile accelerator. Pressure on the pedal causes the automobile and seat to move forward under the driver, which in effect tends to pull the accelerator away from his foot, thus reducing the accelerating force from the engine. This is negative mechanical feedback, and while it could cause a galloping acceleration in a car with excessive power and loose body and seat springing, it usually provides smooth, proportional, self-limiting control that the driver can moderate predictably.

The mechanical problems in steering are no less serious than those in braking, as witness the discontinued Corvair's oversteering problems which are reported to have contributed to so many deaths and injuries (Nader, 1965). Indeed, the hazard in tire failure is a loss of predictable steering ability with such unexpected mechanical feedback characteristics that the driver often cannot compensate soon enough to avert an accident, especially in a turn or on wet pavement, and especially in a small lightweight automobile whose spin speed is faster than that of a longer heavier machine.

The above examples illustrate the nature of good feedback and adverse feedback characteristics that affect a driver's perception of what his machine is doing. We see in Figure 2-1 that his perception is modified by a certain amount of interference entering with the desired information. This may be called *noise* or *static* (as in the case of a weak radio signal). The information that comes back to the driver from his machine should help him to know how well it responds to his commands and what he can expect it to do. Using a stick (machine) to reach a banana is analogous to driving an automobile. Once the stick wielder gets the feel of the char-

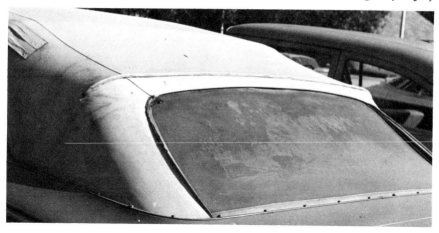

Figure 2-2.   A convertible top with a commonly observed defect in the rear window. This is a severe handicap in backing, parking, changing lanes, and evaluating overtaking traffic.

acteristics of the stick, he uses it as if it were a part of himself. So also the experienced automobile driver knows where each wheel is on the road, what to expect for a certain steering wheel twist or brake push, what an engine miss feels like, when a tire is low, how much room it takes to turn around, and where the bumpers are, just as if these parts of the car were all parts of his own body.

Now let us look at the visual inputs that every driver must have, whether or not he knows his vehicle as an extension of himself. The wide assortment of sources and types of visual information needed and used in driving is indicated in Figure 2-1. The following is a discussion of some of the sources of visual noise that might cause faulty perception and lead to hazardous actions by the driver.

Obstruction of visual input by structural components of the vehicle reduces the information that would be available to the motorist if he were on foot, away from the vehicle. Roof support structures, rear-view mirror, and hood and fenders are the principal obstructors of useful visual information from the driver's seat. (In the case of the hood and fenders, some benefit is provided to the driver by giving real and useful visual cues to his vehicle's size, location, and direction of movement; information that is not supplied in the case of flat-nosed trucks, buses, and vans.) Figures 2-2 through 2-4 show examples of visual obstruction.

The mere presence of a windshield increases the noise level of the visual input. Internal reflections and surface scratch reflections reduce image contrast. Glass surfaces automatically divert by reflection about 20 percent of the visible light (considering a modern windshield set at an

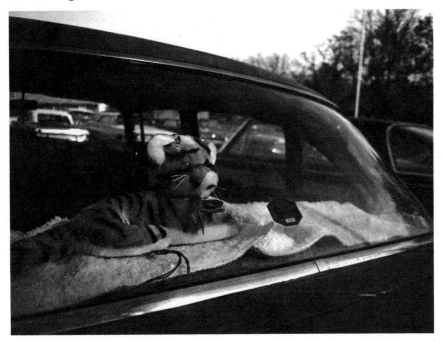

Figure 2-3. This photograph illustrates two problems. The toy with eyes that glow provides some obstruction to rearward view that is probably not very serious. The white rug, which is a common automobile accessory, is of major importance in reducing vision through the rear window. The light from this package shelf, as it is sometimes called, reflects from the glass and gives a veiling luminance over the external scene (much as illustrated in Figure 2-7). Objects pose another hazard when placed in the rear window as illustrated. In the event of a collision they become flying missiles. The package shelf will probably be modified in the future to prevent its use for packages.

angle of 60 degrees from the vertical; see Figure 8-5), and provide a convenient location for dust, water droplets, and bugs to collect. The tinted windshields found in most automobiles cause an additional signal attenuation which effectively raises the noise level. According to the Society of Automotive Engineers (SAE) specifications, a windshield is permitted to lose 30 percent of the visible light at normal incidence. At the actual angle of 60 degrees in the automobile, such a windshield will lose about 39 percent of the visible light. The loss of red light is even greater. At normal incidence, automobile heat-absorbing glass transmits no more than 58 percent of the visible red light. At the 60-degree angle in the automobile, owing to increased filter-path length and increased reflection from the surfaces, only 48 percent of the red end of the spectrum is transmitted. (These figures were derived from Figure 8-9.)

Reflections from windshield surfaces of objects inside the car are a serious source of signal-attenuating noise. The back of a windshield behaves like a mirror, reflecting the top of the dash panel so it appears superimposed on the roadway ahead. If the mirror image of the dash panel top is brighter than the roadway, the motorist finds it difficult to "see through" the reflected image and, in fact, *cannot* see through under certain conditions. See Figures 2-5 through 2-7.

The so-called one-way mirror which allows you to look through at someone without his knowing he is being watched is duplicated quite nicely by the automobile-windshield-dash-panel combination in many automobiles. A one-way mirror has about a 50 percent reflecting surface to-

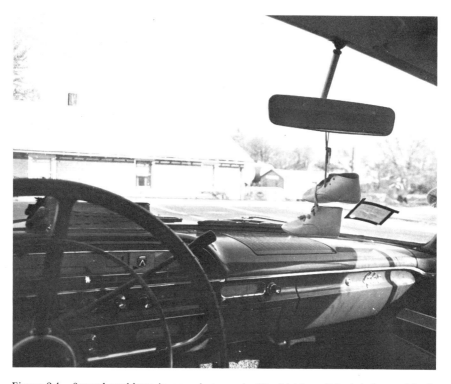

Figure 2-4. Several problems in one photograph. The highly polished dash-panel leads to difficulties (see Figure 2-7); in this case, the old book on the dash-panel top probably gives relief from the glare from the shiny paint. Dangling shoes may be just right to hide a child running into the street. Certainly the dangling motion would mask the presence of a moving automobile on a collision course. If the driver is as short as the position of the camera, the steering wheel would be a significant obstruction to forward vision. If he is tall enough to see over the wheel comfortably, the rear-view mirror would be a large obstruction for objects approaching from the right. Windshield stickers should be banned to avoid their misuse as shown in this photograph. Perhaps the safest place for stickers is the extreme lower left-hand corner as seen from the driver's seat. Other safe positions would be along the bottom of the windshield across in front of the driver to about the midpoint of the car. Such stickers should never be higher than 2 inches or wider than 4 inches.

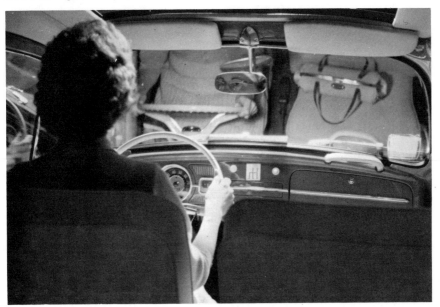

Figure 2-5. A Volkswagen reveals that, with open sun roof, the windows reflect the interior in a way that can be dangerous. An angled windshield reflects only the top of the dash panel, which can be treated to keep the reflections low.

ward the unwitting subject, while the glass itself is a filter, transmitting about 50 percent of the light that gets through the mirrored surface. The one-way mirror only works one way when the amount of light reflected from its mirrored surface is greater than the amount coming through it; hence the viewer must be in a darker room. In the highway scene, objects are often top illuminated or back illuminated so the driver views the shadowed side (the dark room). On the other hand, full sunlight bouncing upward off the top of a light-colored and shiny dash panel will be reflected off the windshield into the driver's eyes. When the reflected light greatly exceeds the light coming from objects on the roadway, presto—the windshield becomes a one-way mirror and roadway objects are obscured.

Oddly enough, the windshield becomes a one-way mirror when viewed from the outside for exactly the same reasons. When you try to look into a car with a tinted windshield, the image of the sky mirrored by the glass is brighter than the light coming from within the car. This phenomenon explains why you often recognize people by their car and not by seeing them within the car—because in many situations this is impossible to do.

Another source of noise typical of automobiles manufactured prior to 1968 is the bright sunlight reflected from chromium surfaces. This noise not only seriously reduces the strength and amount of useful visual

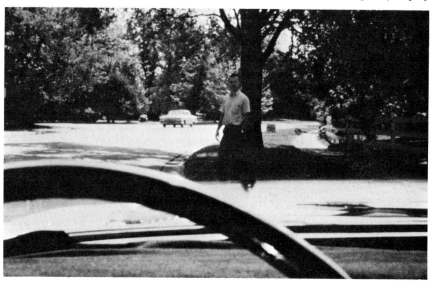

Figure 2-6. Black cloth has been placed over the dash panel to permit vision through this windshield of the pedestrian standing in the shade.

information but also poses an ocular burn hazard to the motorist. We know that we cannot look at the noonday sun for more than a fraction of a minute without causing retinal damage. Polished chromium surfaces reflect upward of 50 percent of the light. If these surfaces are flat or nearly so and of the size of a quarter of a dollar or more held at arm's length, they can reflect enough light into the eye that steady fixation for a minute or more will cause a retinal burn. That retinal burns are not often reported from this cause attests to the fact that a normal person will not or cannot face such glare sources for long. He averts his eyes or closes them for longer than the usual blink period.

The potential for retinal burn points up the intensity that surfaces of polished chromium can provide under certain conditions. High-intensity glare sources have been shown to be visually handicapping, just as one would predict from the nature of the eye and the objects being viewed. Low-intensity large area sources such as a light-colored shiny hood or the sky visible over the roadway also can cause performance losses (Allen, Spring 1968); see Figure 2-8.

The driver is the most important component in the driving task. He must receive and process the information coming to him to eliminate the unimportant and to compensate for the several interferences that occur even under the best conditions. To do this he behaves like a highly sophisticated computer, with a memory bank of experience and training entering into each decision. If he is impaired by alcohol, illness, or other

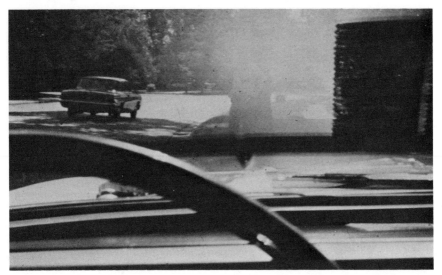

Figure 2-7. View from the same automobile as shown in Figure 2-6 except for removal of the black cloth on the top of the dash panel. The lattice structure to the right is the radio speaker grill. The photographic rendition is not an exaggeration. In fact this photo shows more detail of the wiper structure seen through the steering wheel than Figure 2-6, indicating that an effort was made during printing to bring out the pedestrian's image. Subjectively this situation was uncompensable. The pedestrian could *not* be seen! Improvements have been made in recent automobile production to control glossy reflections from the top of the dash panel. (Indianapolis Star photograph.)

physiologically detrimental factors, the number of events per second that he can process through his computer brain will be proportionately reduced. Heavy traffic increases the number of decisions that must be made and the amount of information that has to be processed. Safe performance with increasing load can be expected only up to a point. Beyond this point the computer driver breaks down, performance becomes erratic, and an accident may ensue.

Speed also increases the perceptual load by requiring that more events per second be processed. Speed reduces the time to think and thus requires greater attention, which is both fatiguing and conducive to errors. A person required to carry on an exciting conversation while driving may become perceptually overloaded at 20 miles per hour; thus, it is difficult to say categorically when perceptual overload begins or whether a given situation constitutes a safe perceptual load. The amount of visual noise, the condition of the driver and of his vehicle, the speed, the traffic density, and the diversions facing the driver must all be considered to determine whether a driver is likely to lose safe control of his vehicle.

The driving task, then, is one of monitoring roadway information visually in the presence of spurious information, signal attenuation, and

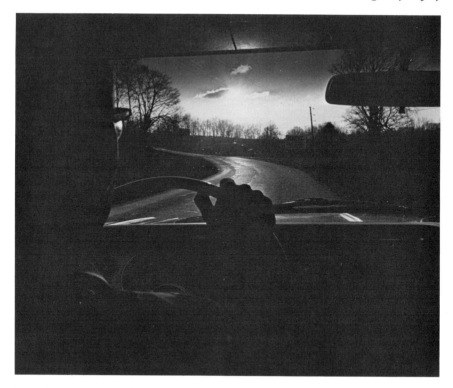

Figure 2-8. Driving against the setting or rising sun causes extreme contrasts. All objects in the scene are seen on the shadowed side while the glare from the sky, clouds, pavement, hood, and windshield dirt may be overpowering. Defects in the windshield are seen in this photo as short lines and small spots of light. Objects on the pavement will be seen in silhouette, but objects off the pavement—for example, the house and fence posts in this picture—are almost impossible to see. A pedestrian might not be seen at all until he stepped onto the bright pavement.

so on, called *noise*. This noisy information is then analyzed against a background of experience and knowledge that is more or less available, depending upon the physiological state and training of the driver. The noise in the visual information is thus analyzed out, and the driver usually perceives a fairly true picture of roadway events, but at a later time. Decisions are made; then motor impulses to the body muscles control the vehicle. The extent to which the vehicle responds is then monitored visually, vestibularly, auditorily, and kinaesthetically. The perceptual time characteristics combined with the driver's reaction time and the time characteristics of the vehicle provide the potential for system oscillation. Such oscillations occur when, for example, an intoxicated person tries to drive. Indeed, the sign of an inexperienced driver is his difficulty in keeping the vehicle going straight and his erratic overcontrol in stops and starts.

Chapter 3: Vision Requirements for Driving

VISUAL ACUITY

GOOD VISUAL ACUITY is the ability to see the fine details of an object at a distance. For a given object, say a person's face, good acuity will allow the recognition of friends, of their facial expressions, and even of their direction of gaze from a great distance. Poorer acuity will be manifest as the need to be closer to an object to recognize its details. In driving, the ability to resolve fine detail permits the reading of signs and signals at a greater distance, thus providing more time in which to change lanes, change speed, or make other maneuvers. Thus, good acuity, 20/20 or better, permits the detection of hazardous situations earlier and provides more time for study and action. The ability of good acuity to provide driving information earlier slows down the action, in effect, and permits the driver to be more relaxed. An acuity of 20/10 would permit twice as much time to act as an acuity of 20/20; with 20/40, only one fourth as much time would be available compared to the excellent 20/10 acuity.

Good acuity implies an optical system that is functioning at top efficiency; night driving visual performance will therefore be best for those with excellent acuity. Similarly, the detection of small objects on the roadway both at night and in the daytime is quickest when good acuity exists. All aspects of vision are usually best when acuity is best; hence the ability of drivers with good acuity should be higher than drivers with poor acuity, all else being equal.

Even though visual acuity is the most easily measured and the most frequently tested for driving, it is a very complex function which is poorly understood. It is inextricably interrelated with contrast, illumination, and exposure duration. If any of the three is reduced, a larger test-letter size is needed. In the automobile, visual acuity is but a small part of the visual requirements for safe driving. It is a central retinal function and cannot be brought into use unless the central retina (fovea centralis retinae) is positioned to receive the image in question. Most images are undoubtedly first noted as being worthy of foveal inspection by peripheral vision.

PERIPHERAL VISION

Those portions of the retina outside the central 5-degree-diameter zone of best acuity are peripheral. The photo receptors in the peripheral retina are less densely packed and have fewer neurons connecting to the brain per unit of retinal area than is the case for the central retina. Numerous important other differences exist; for example, we use the peripheral retina for the majority of our defensive seeing. Any movement within the peripheral field of view of a normal person is instantly detected, and if it is of interest or hazard to us, we will turn our eyes to study the details of the object that moved. All of us have been startled by the unexpected movement of an otherwise unnoticed object in the "corner of our eye." We may jump or scream involuntarily without having had time to fixate the object. It is little realized that accurate information on the spatial direction and distance of objects is obtained from peripheral vision and that a person's own orientation in space is largely a function of the peripheral retina.

The importance of the peripheral retina to driving can be appreciated from the following: We know from eye movement studies that 0.20 to 0.25 seconds are required per fixation. At 60 miles per hour we cover 88 feet of highway per second. With 0.25-second fixations we can inspect the road foveally only at points every 22 feet. The remainder of the scene, with its many details and spatial relationships, must be sensed by peripheral vision. We simply do not have time to inspect every inch of roadway, every tail light, every oncoming car, street sign, or pretty girl, with foveal vision. Without peripheral vision to keep us informed of the big picture and our position within it and to let us know what merits our careful inspection, we would be badly handicapped even for walking around in our own house.

Normal peripheral vision is good but not perfect. For example, in each eye there is a blind area starting about 12 degrees temporalward from the fixation point and covering an oval area about 6 degrees wide and 8 degrees high. There are also numerous sizable blood vessels onto which traffic lights, chuck holes, and even people could be imaged, but where they would not be seen. (Such blind areas are largely compensated for by overlap with good areas in the other eye; the problem is of importance when only one eye is functional.) Furthermore, color vision and visual acuity are reduced in the periphery.

A modern driver cannot afford to be handicapped by defective peripheral vision or by obstructions that might interfere with peripheral vision, caused by such things as vehicle anatomy, spectacle frames, contact lens edge blur, clothing, hair, and hats. Good peripheral vision allows a maximum of information with a minimum of eye movements and hence speeds the detection of hazards or errors in position on the highway. This increased perceptual efficiency allows more time for decision and action by the driver. Good peripheral vision, like good visual acuity, also effectively slows the action in the scene and permits more comfortable and relaxed driving. Freedom from confusion and complete awareness of the driving scene are accompaniments of good peripheral vision.

COLOR VISION

In the modern driving environment red is said to mean stop, yellow to mean danger or caution, and green to mean go. Aside from certain conflicts such as the use of red for advertising, driveway markers, tail lights (not brake lights), Christmas decoration lamps, high-beam indicator lights, and sports car paint, red meaning stop or danger is a reasonable choice. Both red and green are strong signal colors, and traditional usage recommends them for this purpose. However, their use is not without ambiguity and confusion on occasion (Lavender, 1968). The words STOP, CAUTION, and GO in large letters could serve less ambiguously, but the advantage of smaller size and perhaps greater economy lies with the colored signal.

Color coding offers certain real advantages for those with normal color vision. The status of the color vision of the population is that about 0.5 percent of the women and 8 percent of the men have some color vision abnormality. Since aging interferes with color perception because of reduced optical transmission, increased scatter of shorter wavelengths, and neurological deterioration, a higher percentage of apparently defective color vision is to be expected from older people.

Some color vision defects (e.g., deuteranomaly) do not prevent the proper identification of green and red, particularly if the green is bluish. Persons with other defects (protanopia, protanomaly) cannot recognize red except as a light of low intensity, since they are relatively much less sensitive to the longer wavelengths of the spectrum.

Cole et al. (1965) has shown that the color defective driver requires about twice as much time as a normal driver to act upon colored signals, and the incidence of errors in the recognition of the color is much higher. The normal person makes virtually 100 percent correct judgments on red-yellow-green discriminations. Thus the possession of good color vision ensures that practically no mistakes will be made in reading the meaning of red, yellow, and green traffic signals and that they will be read more quickly. Good color vision therefore provides more time in which to make decisions and in effect reduces the perceptual load on the driver. Poor color vision, on the other hand, finds the driver using other clues to try to learn the meaning of a light and, hence, his decisions must always be delayed and uncertain, a circumstance which leads to reduced perceptual capacity and to fatigue.

If we are to continue to license color-defective drivers, they must be advised of the nature of their handicap and the circumstances that must be avoided whenever possible. This presupposes that we know what type of color vision defect is present in a given case. To assist these otherwise usually highly qualified people to drive safely, our signal systems must make allowances for them by providing the information in some way other than by color. Shape coding of signal lights offers a solution. The European highway marker system (see Chapter 10) even uses shape for imparting information that is often written on road signs in the United States.

DARK ADAPTATION

Dark adaptation is the ability of the eyes to increase their sensitivity so that tiny amounts of light are effective in causing visual responses. The measure of the ability to adapt to dark can be either the time required to achieve a given sensitivity level or the level of sensitivity achieved in a given time. Practically, the time in total darkness required for maximum retinal sensitivity to develop is about thirty minutes, although gains in sensitivity may continue to occur over a twenty-four-hour period of total darkness. Sensitivity can rise to such levels that starlight can provide enough light to walk about at night in the open with caution. After five minutes in the dark the rods in the retina become more sensitive than the cones. Rod vision is called *scotopic vision;* cone vision, *photopic vision.* Cones give good acuity and are necessary for color vision. At full moonlight luminance levels the cones are beginning to dominate, and at the luminance levels on the highways the cones are definitely dominant. Adaptation to night highway luminance levels is reasonably complete within five minutes in the dark, and adaptation to the fluctuations in luminance of objects on the roadway occurs within a few seconds.

Most people adapt quickly to the levels of nighttime highway luminance. Individual differences show up best only after total dark adaption for twenty-five to thirty minutes, a condition never encountered on the modern highway. However, older drivers with small pupils and/or incipient cataracts have reduced ocular transmission, and thus their retinal luminance levels may be one fifth to one twentieth of normal. Night road luminance levels would be too low for such people to use photopic vision; hence their overall visual performance would be significantly inferior to that of younger drivers. Drivers with retinal pathology or with neurological involvements are also likely to suffer from an abnormal loss of visual performance at night highway luminance levels.

Testing for impaired ability to see at night should be done routinely, especially on those persons of advanced age and with known retinal pathology. A test with a low luminance background such as the Night Vision Performance Tester (Allen and Lyle, Nov. 1963) would give an indication of the person's ability to perform at low luminance levels.

GLARE RESISTANCE

The ability to recognize useful information in a visual display in the presence of a bright source of light is called *glare resistance*. The ability to resist glare is an individual characteristic dependent upon a variety of factors, almost all of which degrade the quality of the optical image falling on the photoreceptors. The better the optical system is, the better it will behave in the presence of glare. Sometimes neurological and retinal factors, usually pathological, can be such that glare (overexcitation) at some point in the field of view will cause an overall reduction in visual performance. Whatever the factors, the better the visual system behaves in the presence of a glare source, the greater is said to be its glare resistance.

At night on the highway the driver faces approaching headlights at the same time that he is required to see roadway details well enough to avoid hazards and remain on his own portion of the road. This is the classic concept of why a driver needs good glare resistance and why he should be tested for glare resistance. While glare is often thought of in terms of distress caused by oncoming headlights at night, it also enters into a normal daytime scene where no glare sources in the accepted sense are present (Allen, Spring 1968). When an optical system scatters light, the scattered light reduces the contrast of all images on the retina and thus reduces visual performance. It is common experience that glare resistance becomes significantly greater when a lens correction is supplied to eliminate refractive errors. Thus, the eye with poor glare resistance may also be an eye with poor image quality.

Under conditions of high luminances with good shadow detail, no difficulties in operating a motor vehicle would be expected even though glare resistance is low. At low luminances, on the other hand, especially at twilight or on dull days when no shadows are present to accentuate objects, the visual performance on the highway will be impaired if glare resistance is low. At night, of course, the ability to see the roadway may be severely impaired if glare resistance is low. Interestingly, the average automobile windshield adds so much stray light, due to scratches, pits, internal reflections, and dirt, both in the daytime and at night, that the driving glare resistance of even the most glare-resistant individual, as tested in the license bureau, will be inadequate to permit safe operation of the vehicle at night. In other words, it is probably academic to worry about the glare resistance of the driver himself when we exercise no control over smoke-stained windshields that have 50,000 miles of wiper scratches, plus abrasions from service station cleaning, in addition to the variable collection of dirt and water droplets found on the outside of the glass. Fortunately it seems that those mostly older drivers who have poor glare resistance and dark adaptation tend to limit themselves to driving only during the hours of daylight; however, there is no way to ensure that the automobiles on the roads at night have clean new windshields.

REACTION TIME

The time to respond to stimulus, such as a flash of light, given to a person who has been instructed to push a switch as soon as he can, is called his *reaction time*. It involves photochemical, neurological, and perhaps psychological delays on the sensory side and neurological, muscular, switch, and timer delays on the motor side. Classically the fastest one can expect a response to a visual stimulus is about 0.18 second. Older people react more slowly, as do people in poor health. Complex situations cause longer reaction times. The usual reaction time to a red brake or stop light in controlled experiments on the highway is about 0.55 second in alert responsive subjects. About twice as long is required for color defectives, and still longer when weaker stimuli are used.

The factors affecting reaction times are both optical and physiological. A person whose central nervous system is depressed by alcohol, barbiturates, carbon monoxide, or lipemia (a high blood cholesterol level), will have a longer reaction time. A person receiving weak stimuli will take longer to react; hence those with small pupils, an absorptive or a scattering optical media, or a pair of dark-tinted sun glasses can expect a significantly longer reaction time.

A person driving at today's speeds and densities of traffic must be able to make decisions quickly and accurately. Modern highway driving demands are becoming so great that slow-responding drivers are indeed a hazard. Slow response often means slow thinking and inadequate understanding of the hazards. One really ought not to laugh at such jokes as the one defining a split second as the time between the light change and the honking of the horn of the car in back. There are great differences in driver alertness and ability to react to a hazardous situation.

A visual reaction time test should be given to drivers applying for license and license renewal because of its ability to measure the performance of the whole driver. In fact, incorporating a visual reaction time tester into every automobile dash panel would be an excellent means of warning a motorist when his overall functional ability is impaired. He may need to use a pair of glasses, or to sober up, or to get off the road if he has been driving too long or has been exposed to noxious fumes.

OCULAR MUSCLE IMBALANCE

Ocular muscle imbalance, currently largely ignored in driver tests, probably is an important contributor to driver inefficiency. In-, out-, or upturning tendencies (eso-, exo-, or hyperphorias) are usually more or less easily compensated for by a driver at normal daytime levels of illumination, although the effort to compensate may take its toll in fatigue and discomfort. On the other hand, at night a little imbalance may become unmanageable, the more so if the driver is fatigued, overfed or drugged —as by alcohol, carbon monoxide, or medications. When a tendency to turn the eyes is uncompensated, double vision results. Double vision of sudden onset can be catastrophic, especially to a naïve driver. I believe that a large proportion of the one-car accidents late at night result from misjudgments by young drivers who have 0.75 diopter or more of uncorrected hyperopia and who are fatigued. Upon loss of the bright lights of other cars, as happens late at night, they may lose control of fusion, lapse into a crossed-eye condition, become confused and frightened, and run off the road. Such youngsters typically have 20/20 vision or better in the daytime.

Darkness tends to cause an accommodative in-turning of the eyes (esophoria) to about the plane of the windshield, even in normal eyes. In many situations windshield dirt or water can be a stronger fusion stimulus than the highway proper, thus causing the eyes to turn in and the road to be seen double. Certainly a test for hyperopia and muscle imbalance should be a mandatory part of a license bureau eye test, and some information about the hazards of driving late at night should be given to the farsighted youngster with good acuity.

Chapter 4: Space Perception and Driving

THE PROBLEM

WITHOUT adequate space perception, good visual acuity, color vision, dark adaptation, and fields of vision are not enough to permit safe driving. It is believed that the development of space perception is largely learned and requires a long time of dynamic interaction with one's environment. Those human beings who at an early age have done the normal amounts of running, jumping, throwing, climbing, and chasing, will have a reasonably good appreciation of space. If these early experiences were not normal because of such things as illness, congenital cataracts, or the need for a pair of glasses, the appreciation of spatial relationships will not be as good, thereby constituting a degree of handicap for driving. Those, for example, who "couldn't hit the side of a barn" when throwing a ball are probably not muscularly defective, as often believed, but rather perceptually defective, being unable to accurately localize objects in the space around them. The person who cannot park without occasionally creasing a fender, or who parks two feet away from the curb or strikes the curb hard in angle parking, or hugs the center line in driving, or bumps the garage door, probably is a person with a space perception problem. Such little problems become critical problems when high speeds and long-distance judgments are involved.

Alcohol is an example of a judgment-impairing and spatially disorienting agent, and alcohol is now credited with being involved in over 50 percent of all fatal accidents (Selzer and Weiss, 1966). New drivers who have not developed good spatial judgment in the driving task have the highest accident rates of all drivers, whether they are in their teens or in their forties. Deceptive arrangement of some of the clues to space perception have been demonstrated to have marked effects upon the judgment and stopping distances of drivers (Allen and Crosley, May 1967). Thus the evidence grows that adequate clues to space perception and adequate skill in interpreting those clues are essential to safe motoring.

Space perception is almost entirely relative, which accounts for the

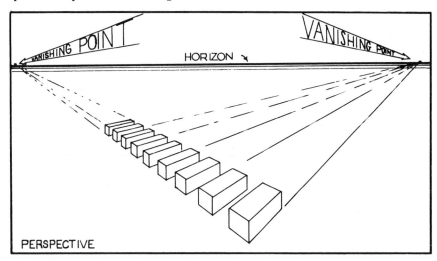

Figure 4-1. The visual angle of an object becomes smaller with increasing distance. This is unconsciously interpreted as a distance change and not a size change. Thus we see objects as if they were of the same angular size but at different distances. This drawing shows how vanishing points may be used in drawing a scene.

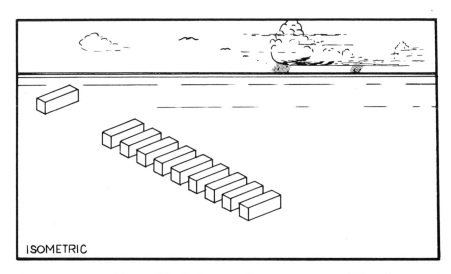

Figure 4-2. When objects of identical sizes are drawn into a scene which makes some of them appear farther away, the conflict in size and distance is resolved by interpreting the distance about right and the size as increasing with greater distance. The block house at the left is of course, identical in measured size to the one at the right. This illusion is based upon the fact that an object is judged to be farther away if it is higher in the scene; that is, nearer to the horizon.

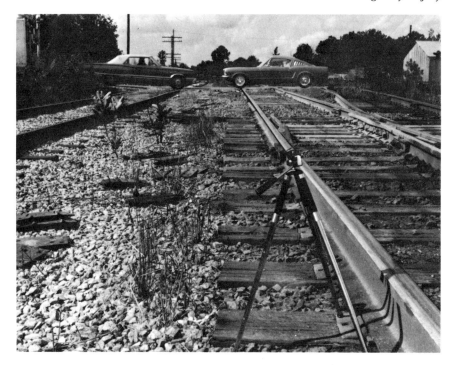

Figure 4-3. Two automobiles appear to be on a collision course. However, one subtle clue is the absence of a shadow under the Mustang. See Figure 4-4.

ease with which we can be fooled in our judgments of speed, location, and direction of movement of vehicles, including our own. There are both monocular and binocular clues available to the driver, which he uses unconsciously. The following discussion will show the complexity of the information supplied to the driver and will clarify the need for the driver to be in good health, sober, and possessed of extensive experience in making highway space judgments.

PERSPECTIVE CLUES

Railroad tracks appear to diminish to a point on the horizon because of the diminishing angular subtense of an object at greater distances. The object-image relationship in cameras and eyes is such that for a given focus-setting the image size is inversely proportional to the object distance. Hence the farther away the railroad track, the smaller is its image. Equal-sized objects will be imaged equally in size only if they are at equal distances from the observer.

The human brain does not interpret different retinal image sizes of

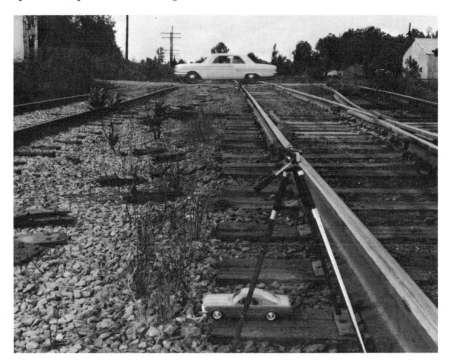

Figure 4-4. When the Mustang is removed from its wire frame atop the tripod and placed at the foot of the tripod, its true size becomes apparent. Or put another way, its actual size has not changed much but the judgment of its distance has been greatly modified by lowering it to the surface of the ground. The lesson is clear. For an object to be accurately localized and correctly judged for size and shape, it must be visibly attached to or rest upon the ground or pavement. (The measured small decrease in physical size in this photograph compared to Figure 4-3 is owing to the increased distance from the lens of the camera when the model sits on the ground.)

similar objects as different-sized objects, but rather as equal-sized objects at different distances. This is possible by judging the object relative to other objects in the field of view, using perspective clues.

Figure 4-1 shows a simple scene with vanishing points for the main lines in the surfaces. Figure 4-2 shows the effect of ignoring perspective clues in part of the drawing. Size constancy is the ability of a person to judge that a distant object is the same size as a nearby one or, said another way, the ability to relate loss in image size to increased distance and not to an object shrinkage. Without relative positioning in a scene, errors of judgment of size and position are common. A normally proportioned but small object will be interpreted as farther away than it really is, even though the position within the scene should accurately locate it. Figures 4-3 and 4-4 illustrate that, when placed high, near the horizon, the small car looks big and far away. When placed lower in the scene, its diminished size is apparent because it is localized nearby. This is one of the principal perspective clues: that more distant objects are usually nearer the level of the horizon. When an object is exactly at eye level (horizon height), this location clue is lost. Then only its image size and the memory of its true size are of help in localizing it.

A useful indicator of relative distance on the highway is overlay, or the obliteration of part of one object by another object which is nearer.

ATMOSPHERIC CLUES

An important clue to distance is provided by atmospheric effects upon transmitted light. These effects are atmospheric boil, attenuation, and scatter. Their action, singly or in combination, is a tendency to reduce contrast, to reduce border sharpness, to attenuate and shift colors toward the red, and to make blues look black. Superimposed over these effects is additional scattered blue light, which increases with distance until the object cannot be seen and only a blue haze remains.

Atmospheric boil results when air is heated, becomes turbulent, and thus presents multiple and varying refractive index irregularities throughout its volume; this makes distant objects shimmer. Shimmering is usually so rapid that in effect it blurs the borders of objects. The amount of shimmer increases with distance.

Atmospheric attenuation and scatter are related to each other and to distance. Objects that appear to be less bright are thus associated with being farther away. Loss of color of familiar objects and the presence of a veiling blue haze clearly are associated with great distance.

ILLUMINATION CLUES

Brightness, especially at night, is a major clue to distance, partly because there are few others. When an object is far enough away that it subtends about 1 minute of arc (3.5 inches at 1,000 feet), further increase in its distance causes no change in point image size but rather causes a loss in retinal image illumination per unit area in compliance with the inverse square law; that is, twice the distance reduces the light on the retina to one fourth. For people with 20/40 acuity, the critical size is 2 minutes or 3.5 inches at 500 feet. Thus, past experience leads us to believe that dim points of light are farther away than bright ones, though they are at exactly the same distance. Errors in judgment are regularly made when judging small lights at a distance; for example, in one test red tail lights at 270 feet were judged to be much farther away than white lights at 750 feet.

Larger sources such as automobile surfaces or signs do not lose brightness with ordinary driving distances, except for atmospheric losses. They must be very far away to subtend 1 minute of angle or less at the observer's eye.

STEREOPSIS OR BINOCULAR PARALLAX

Stereopsis is considered to be the highest skill of a person with binocular vision. It is the relative judgment of spatial relationships dependent only upon the subtle differences in view provided by the separation of the two eyes. If the eyes are properly oriented, split-second exposures of the two eyes simultaneously is enough to provide stereo awareness of spatial relationships. Stereopsis is relative and depends upon a framework of known objects for accurate localization. Stereoscopic range finders have great accuracy, but the observer is asked merely to equate the distances of a fixed reticle and the target in question. The accuracy of the instrument depends upon how accurately it projects the fixed reticle into the scene.

Stereopsis is a powerful help in localization of objects within a person's immediate environment, such as at his work bench. Since all space judgments are relative, it is important that the observer know exactly where some of the objects in his environment are at all times. By touching or handling nearby objects, an absolute reference for judging more remote objects by stereopsis and other clues is provided. A person who must attempt several times to grasp a pencil or a control knob has faulty stereopsis and cannot be expected to perform well on tasks where monocular clues to space perception are largely absent, as in driving a car at night. One-eyed people have a real handicap in spatial perception, as they are dependent entirely upon the several monocular clues, which may sometimes be absent and at best will require more time to interpret. A person without stereopsis is essentially one-eyed and is at least as handicapped in space perception as the one-eyed person.

MONOCULAR PARALLAX

When a person moves his head, visual objects shift their relative positions within the scene. This shift due to head movement is called *monocular parallax*. One may move his head, move himself, or be in a moving vehicle. The term monocular is used to differentiate it from binocular parallax, which is stereopsis or a simultaneous comparison of the different views for the two eyes. Monocular parallax causes near objects to appear to move against the movement of the observer while remote objects move with the observer. The relative speed of object movement is related to the distance of the object from a reference object, the speed of observer movement, and the distance of the observer from the reference object.

The ability to make parallactic judgments is very good. Movement of a sizable object within a scene can be detected when it moves more than 6 minutes of arc when viewing conditions are good. This requires an object of good contrast in a detailed environment and a movement that is completed in a short period of time. Hazard exists when no monocular parallax occurs as a result of real movement of the object itself. When an object is on a collison course with a car, it grows in size and does not change its direction from the driver. Hence a collision course with its disastrous termination is devoid of monocular parallax clues and as a result is the most difficult to detect.

VELOCITY JUDGMENTS

In collision situations the only clue to the hazard is the increasing size of the object. If seen early, an intuitive guess by the driver that a collision is imminent may be made. The ability to judge an increase in size is a function of the distance and the object. Halving the distance doubles the size. A car traveling at 60 miles per hour covers half a mile in thirty seconds. It doubles its size in thirty seconds if it is first noted one mile away. Assuming it is about 7.25 feet wide, its angular size will have increased from 5 minutes to 10 minutes of arc. For comparison, a 20/20 letter subtends 5 minutes of arc. Imagine it requiring thirty seconds to grow to a 20/40 letter size! Such slow size changes at great distances cannot mean much. On the other hand it only takes fifteen seconds for the size to double again as the car travels from 0.5 to 0.25 mile away. As the car approaches, doubling in apparent size occurs at increasingly shorter intervals and the angular size rapidly increases. For example, in traveling from 200 feet to 100 feet the size will double in just 1.13 seconds. The angular increase will be from 125 to 250 minutes of arc, while the area increase would be proportional to the square of these numbers. Thus, it is difficult to judge the speed of an approaching automobile until the rate of its angular size change exceeds the threshold value for a given individual.

Judgment of closing speed is a function of vehicle size, distance, and rate of travel. Trucks would seem to approach faster than regular cars, which would seem faster than compact or sports cars or motorcycles. A motorist will usually not pass when faced by an approaching truck even though there is adequate time. On the other hand, he may elect to pass when faced by a motorcycle or low-slung sports car when inadequate passing time exists. In general, the changing angular size is of little value for judging a vehicle's speed when it is more than 1,000 feet away.

Chapter 5: Vision Tests

THE COMPLETE optometric examination will be outlined, and those areas of particular concern in vision tests for drivers will be discussed in detail. It is assumed that the reader of this chapter has a basic proficiency in making the tests so that the remarks can be directed to refinements in clinical testing and special precautions that may not be generally understood. This chapter is not directed toward the needs of the license bureau tester or legislator, although certain portions could be of general informational value.

The complete visual and ocular examination, sometimes referred to as the "21-point" examination, is outlined as follows:

A. Case History: An exploration of the following areas by interrogation
   1. Chief complaint of patient
   2. Nature of work, lighting, distances, etc., associated with patient's job
   3. Patient's statement of symptoms or history of disease, both ocular and systemic
   4. Medications, internal or external, currently being taken by patient
   5. Extent of use of alcohol and tobacco by the patient
   6. Environmental chemical exposure of patient, both at home and at work
   7. Scintillating scotoma and migraine headaches
B. Preliminary Examination: A search for pathology or abnormality
   1. Visual acuity test
   2. Motility of eyes
   3. Visual fields test
   4. Pupil dynamics and the iris
   5. Lids and cornea
   6. Lens and vitreous clarity
   7. Fundus study

        8. Intraocular pressure measurements
        9. Photomyoclonic, photoconvulsive, and photophobic tendencies
    C. Refraction
        1. Objective Tests
        2. Subjective Tests
            a. monocular
            b. binocular
    D. Five Fundamental Variables of Ocular Muscle Coordination
        1. Distance phoria
        2. Positive fusional convergence
        3. Negative fusional convergence
        4. Amplitude of accommodation
        5. A.C.A. ratio
    E. Special Tests
        1. Aniseikonia
        2. Color vision
        3. Stereopsis
        4. Night visual performance
        5. Visual fields
        6. Reaction time
        7. Glaucoma

CASE HISTORY

If given the opportunity by an attentive examiner, the patient will tell what his major symptoms are and what he wants done. Through careful sympathetic questioning, most of the information needed about health, medication, diet, and intoxicants becomes readily available. Specific questions about driving should be asked, including what make and model automobile, the color of the hood and dash-panel top, and the location of chromium surfaces that can reflect the sky. Ask about seeing double at night, such as occurs by double reflection within the windshield. Ask if he wears sunglasses to drive; if so, take a look at them. They should not be clip-overs and should not be green or made of wavy glass or plastic. Ideally they should be gray polarizing with prescription incorporated, with large lenses that tend to "wrap around" and with thin frames and high temples.

Ask if he wears night-driving glasses of any kind; if so, inspect them. They should not be tinted any color including yellow, except for the lightest shades of cosmetic pink. Green sunglasses, tinted windshields, and Thermanon all absorb red excessively and are not recommended for any driving day or night.

Does the patient have trouble seeing street signs at night; seeing against headlight glare; seeing with normal amounts of light in the home, in the yard at night, and so forth? Problems here can indicate increasing ocular scatter, as in a beginning cataract; the steamy cornea of glaucoma; increased light absorption; or pinhole pupils, both of which reduce the light available on the retina; or they may indicate a systemic problem which interferes with retinal metabolism, such as a vitamin deficiency or the presence of toxic agents harmful to the retina or neural pathways. So simple and common a toxic agent as carbon monoxide interferes with dark adaptation, accommodation, and fusion, while chronic alcoholism or inadequate diet may cause a deficiency of vitamin A.

Drugs of interest to inquire about are those that cause pupil constriction and accommodative activity (parasympathomimetic), paralysis of accommodation and dilation of the pupil (parasympatholytic), or dilation of the pupil alone (sympathomimetic). The *Physicians' Desk Reference* or equivalent will provide needed information on the effects of a particular drug the patient is using. The *Merck Manual* will provide information on what drugs are commonly used for what diseases. This will assist whenever the patient is unaware of what medication he is taking but knows the name of his disease.

Information on smoking is of two-fold interest. If the patient is a smoker of cigarettes about which he has repeatedly been warned, you know he has little regard for himself; he is also apt to be a less safe driver because of his attitude (Adams and Williams). The second reason for interest in smoking is that tobacco smoke contains carbon monoxide, and the street and highway atmospheres have significant levels of carbon monoxide as well. The effect of carbon monoxide is exaggerated by altitude and alcohol and principally consists of anoxia at the tissue level. Anoxia causes "red-out" and, finally, "black-out" when it occurs in the head region, just as positive G forces cause these same symptoms in an aircraft pilot. Accommodation is impaired, esophoria occurs, fusional amplitudes fall, and 0.50 to 1.50 diopters of accommodative myopia may occur. Asthenopia, diplopia, blurring, headache, and drowsiness can all result from smoking by itself or smoking combined with high levels of atmospheric carbon monoxide. In addition, the dark-adaptation ability is impaired and the recovery from bright headlights will be delayed.

The need to know about environmental intoxicants is of great importance for similar reasons. Many people do not realize that lead absorbed from food, drink, and air amounts to 30 micrograms a day in the city for an average nonsmoker and 40 for a smoker. This can lead to symptoms of lead poisoning, especially if other exposures occur. Gasoline, carbon tetrachloride, and many other chemical vapors common around the house and job can be detrimental to health. Hair sprays, hair dyes, perfumes, tooth paste, and other "harmless" items can cause trouble for some people. Symptoms often mimic eye disorders or cause eye changes. Two classical examples are naphthalene (moth balls), which cause ingestion or long exposure to the vapors can cause cataract, and insecticides, which may cause accommodative spasms as well as wide systemic problems. Moth crystals, toilet and room deodorizers, insecticides, and cleaning solvents are common in many homes, with little thought being given to their hazardous nature. There are many other cataractogenic and systemically toxic chemicals that a workman may encounter on his job or a do-it-yourself artist may expose himself to. They are all the more hazardous in spray-can form.

The use of atropine and related drugs is widespread. Atropine and related alkaloids are poisons that have medicinal value. They have a parasympatholytic action, their effects are cumulative, and they require about two weeks to wear off. These alkaloids are available without a prescription in cold remedies (such as Contac), laxatives (Alophen Pills), rectal suppositories (Wyanoids), and asthma powders (Asthamador), among others. They and related compounds are regularly and freely prescribed for intestinal, digestive, and ulcer symptoms and to dry up mucous secretions. The effect of small doses over prolonged periods of time by self-medication or by prescription will most assuredly be worse than the ill it was intended to treat. Typical symptoms are blurring of vision because of enlarged pupils and a paralysis of accommodation, dryness of the eyes, and asthenopia due to a higher than normal A.C.A. ratio. Vague symptoms of eye distress, pain, and headache may be due to atropine-caused elevated intraocular pressure. Certainly it is well known that atropine is a provocative test for glaucoma, yet apparently it is little realized that atropine anywhere in the body affects the eyes if ingested long enough. One interesting clue to atropine poisoning is male impotence!

Extensive use of alcohol is harmful to the liver, which is the important reservoir of vitamin A needed by the eyes. Tobacco-alcohol amblyopia appears to be due almost entirely to vitamin deficiencies. Night blindness and xerophthalmia with eventual corneal opacification is the result of prolonged vitamin A deficiency. The effects of alcohol in some ways resemble carbon monoxide poisoning. The ability of alcohol to remove social inhibitions also seems to parallel losses of inhibitory behavior of visual pathways because border contrasts, successive contrasts, and hence acuity and threshold visibilities are degraded. The increased reaction times and general disorientation of the "drunk," especially at night, make him, as statistics have shown, a poor risk on the highway, either as a driver or a pedestrian.

A record of a person's visual symptoms without pertinent questions about poisons, drugs, intoxicants, and nutrients is apt to prove misleading when one attempts to determine whether spectacles will relieve the symptoms.

Scintillating scotomas and migraine headaches have been the subjects of many papers and studies. Generally they are considered to be of little importance, and treatment is often only symptomatic. On the assumption that these phenomena are the result of vascular disturbances, the author has found experimental evidence that niacin, a B vitamin, taken in a 50- to 100-mg. dose at the first prodromal visual symptoms, will, in a high percentage of cases, halt the development of the scintillating scotomas and avert the headache that normally follows the visual disturbances. Recent medical evidence indicates that natural and induced migraine attacks can be aborted by increasing the level of serotonin in the system. During the height of the untreated scintillation phenomena, the retina has very poor sensitivity in the portions of the visual field affected and may become completely blind for a short time. Since the scintillation effect usually starts as a small area in the periphery and grows over a ten- or fifteen-minute period to include a major portion of the field, often sparing the fovea, the patient has adequate warning of the impending visual disability.

If relief medication is not at hand, the driver should not continue driving until after the scotomas have entirely disappeared. Even then the migraine headache that usually follows would probably make driving unwise. A person with a history of migraine or scintillating scotoma should be studied carefully to determine whether a refractive error, aniseikonia, muscle imbalance, or incoordination could be contributing factors. Since many migraine patients have all but given up hope of obtaining relief from their malady, they may not know that relief can sometimes be dramatic. They should be referred, when indicated, for further medical consideration and treatment.

PRELIMINARY EXAMINATION

Visual Acuity Test

This portion of the optometric examination is a search for pathology and for hereditary, traumatic, or functional anomalies. The first test is visual acuity. While there are many factors that affect visual acuity, the test does give an indication of the visual efficiency at the test distance and for the test illumination. A valuable aid to visual acuity testing would be an acuity chart with luminance variable from 150 down to 0.5 apparent foot-candles. The Night Vision Performance Tester (Allen and Lyle, 1963) provides a suitably wide range of luminances, in addition to providing low-contrast visual acuity targets which simplify the assessment of reductions in visual performance due to ametropia, abnormal pupil size, ocular scatter, and absorption in the ocular media. It is certain that an acuity of 20/40 at high luminances will deteriorate, perhaps to less than 20/200, at night roadway luminances (Allen and Lyle, 1963; Richards, May 1966). Adjustment of luminance on a specific target, from too low upward until the target is just readable, provides a sensitive test for evaluating the effects of small lens-power changes or small changes in cataract density.

MOTILITY OF EYES

Ocular motility needs to be tested in all quadrants of the fixation field to determine whether a paresis or paralysis exists. Equally important is to watch the eyes track a moving target. An eye movement record may be taken with the American Optical Company Ophthalmograph (no longer manufactured), the Education Development Laboratory eye movement camera (Taylor, 1960), the direct writing Eye-Trac Camera,* or the eye movement camera using Polaroid film developed by the author.† An eye movement camera is to the vision specialist what the X-ray machine is to the dentist. A significant percentage of people are visually poorly coordinated. The result of general uncoordination or poor ocular coordination is easy disorientation, frequent errors of judgment, and ease of confusion, none of which is desirable while climbing stairs, walking across a street, or driving an automobile.

The value of testing for gross visual uncoordinations is that something can and should be done for it. The beauty of using an eye movement camera is that, once accomplished, the improved coordination can be recorded, measured, and shown to the patient, who will probably also have noticed a favorable difference in his visual comfort and confidence. Gross motor coordination tests give information about the visuomotor coordination and should be included whenever case history, examination results, or recent accident experience indicates a need. High degrees of esophoria or exophoria at distance are unusual, fortunately, but they should not be accepted as unchangeable and should not be allowed to stand when the patient is likely to do any driving at night. Prism correction may work, provided ghost images from lens internal reflections do not negate their benefit. Visual training or rehabilitation can modify phorias favorably and, combined with spectacles, can make a comfortable and safer nighttime driver.

If a paresis is present, much improvement or even complete compensation can be achieved with visual therapy. If a paralysis exists, often enough rehabilitation work can be done to allow comfortable binocular vision in at least a portion of the visual field. An eye that has had muscle surgery will almost always show abnormalities of coordination and of muscle fields. Such eyes have been injured, and visual rehabilitation is needed just as surely as it is after facial and ocular injuries in an automobile crash. Such people should be studied carefully to see if it is safe or can be made safe for them to operate a motor vehicle at night.

* Eye-Trac Direct Reading Eye Movement Monitor, Biometrics, Inc., 40 Ames Street, Cambridge, Mass., 02142.

† Supported by the American Optometric Foundation Motorists' Night Vision Grant to Indiana University.

VISUAL FIELDS TEST

A number of authors have shown that glaucoma symptoms will appear in the central visual fields (tangent screen) virtually every time there is a peripheral field restriction; hence, peripheral fields would not seem to be more valuable than central fields for glaucoma study. For this reason it is desirable that a multiple-pattern visual field screening device be used on every patient regardless of age. The confrontation test is crude but often quite adequate to pick up extreme peripheral field lesions. For drivers the horizontal limits to the visual field should be run on a perimeter or a screening device similar to those used in driver licensing bureaus and driver training schools, such as the Porto-Clinic. Any loss in visual fields to less than 180 degrees is abnormal and is cause for suspicion of pathology. The driving limitation in some states of not less than 140 degrees of horizontal visual field is purely an arbitrary cut-off point for driver testing. A person with only 140 degrees of visual field has some kind of abnormality which may be in the retina, central neurology, or optics of the eye (usually lenticular). It may also be due to the field limitations in a pair of cataract or even standard spectacles!

Since peripheral vision is essential to driving an automobile safely, any field anomaly should be evaluated as to its dangerous effects on driving. Even a reduction in the color fields for red and amber may be sufficient grounds for advising against driving. Fields are of little value unless taken through an adequate correction lens. Ametropia and/or presbyopia must be corrected. The newer tangent-screen-type testing machines make testing and recording of visual field defects both easy and fast and are highly recommended. Careful adherence to target size, brightness standards, and surround brightnesses is essential for repeatable results.

PUPIL DYNAMICS AND THE IRIS

The pupil can be a useful source of information to the examiner. A large pupil will predispose to higher retinal illuminations, and most pupils open wide at night. Since the pupil musculature is both sympathetically and parasympathetically innervated, it can show the systemic effects of sympathomimetic and parasympathomimetic agents. It also mirrors the effects of emotions, accommodation, convergence, light, mental activity, glaucoma, iritis, and neurological lesions. It even appears that abnormal binocular vision may cause an abnormal pupil size of one or both pupils.

An anisocoria which produces a two-to-one difference in image intensity between the two eyes will cause significant visual space perception anomalies (Lit, 1966). Greater differences can occur as, for example, in the early stages of monocular cataract formation with its increased light absorption in the one lens. Patients with image intensity differences between the two eyes will be confused by rapidly moving objects in the

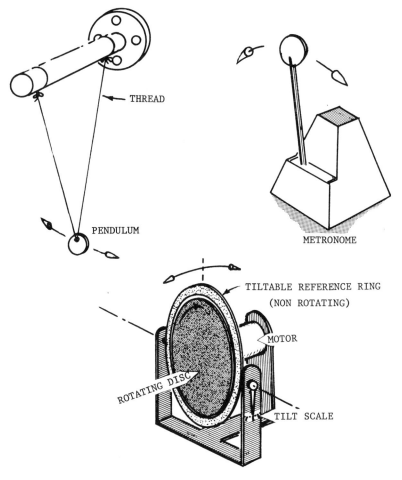

DEVICES FOR EQUATING RETINAL ILLUMINATION

Figure 5-1. Three methods for demonstrating the Pulfrich stereo effect. All involve a moving target and a difference in luminance levels at the two retinas, as by a filter before one eye.

field of view. The phenomenon is called the Pulfrich stereo effect.

Measurements of pupil size may not reveal the existence of a Pulfrich stereo anomaly because it may be due to absorption in the lens, to different f-values of each eye, to the presence of a neurological anomaly, or even to a blurred uniocular image which then behaves like a reduced intensity image. When any doubt exists, it is wise to test for the anomaly. Testing of course is unnecessary if the patient does not have good binocular vision with stereopsis. Figure 5-1 shows a white pendulum which will move in a plane and be seen correctly by the normal patient. It will be seen to move in an ellipse by the person with unequal optical image intensities, with a lowered monocular border gradient due to ametropia or ocular scatter, or even with difference in image size.

Figure 5-1 also shows the use of a metronome for testing the relative luminances of the retinas of the two eyes. A larger excursion can be obtained by casting a shadow of the moving disc on a translucent screen or on a large projection screen. The third device, a tiltable-ring rotating-disc apparatus, offers a precise means of measuring these effects (Walker, 1968) or of balancing the two eyes by eliminating the tilt of the moving disc.

LIDS AND CORNEA

Lids, cilia, and the palpebral conjunctiva should be healthy and in normal relationship to the eyes. Evidences of chronic or acute inflammation are an adequate basis for referral. Corneal hazing, epithelial edema, or purulent material in the tear fluid are all contributory to increased ocular scatter and to poor night vision in particular. In addition such inflammation of the lids and conjunctiva may be symptomatic of vitamin A deficiency, which is important in nighttime seeing. The cilia in an older person may turn in toward the cornea and account for photophobic symptoms, tearing, and asthenopia. The cilia may be absent or not dense and dark enough to form a sun shade to help reduce sky glare, thus contributing to photophobia. On the other hand, they may droop so low that they split the pupil into multiple pinholes, thus causing all manner of weird symptoms. There is some evidence that eyelash cosmetics flake off and enter the eye, causing corneal abrasions similar to those from wearing contact lenses and thus producing photophobic symptoms. Hair sprays can also be a problem, especially for contact lens wearers. Exposure to ultraviolet light, as in snow fields, at high altitudes, in welding, over the water, in the laboratory, or under a sun lamp, will cause a painful burn of the corneal epithelium which, when severe, is called *snow blindness*. An ultraviolet burn is characterized by extreme photophobia. Iritis and uveitis are also characterized by photophobic symptoms. The post-surgical cataract patient suffers photophobia also, because of the increased ocular transmission and the increase in the effective f-number of the eye-spectacle-lens combination.

LENS AND VITREOUS CLARITY

The lens and vitreous contribute much of interest to the patient's symptoms. Excessive scattering and losses in transmission are usually lenticular in origin. Sometimes the cornea or vitreous or even the retina itself may be implicated in the intraocular scatter of light. The healthy cornea seems never to cloud up (Allen and Vos, 1967) even up to age eighty. Corneal clouding is usually indicative of glaucoma, vitamin deficiency, or interstitial keratitis. The lens, on the other hand, shows progressive deterioration of optical clarity from the earliest stages. The B vitamins, with good nutrition, seem to offer some hope of delaying or reversing the aging of the crystalline lens. Some encouraging results have been observed in improving ocular transmission and reducing lens opacity in selected cases with proteolytic enzymes. Since these substances may have some hazard, studies are proceeding cautiously. The vitreous remains clear unless uveitis or retinitis exists. Vitreous floaters, however, accompany liquification of the vitreous and are generally thought to be untreatable. Three points of interest are (1) the floaters are more conspicuous when a small pupil exists, (2) the floaters may pose less of a problem or disappear altogether after the patient improves his nutrition and health, and (3) quick and large eye movements can often displace a large floater away from the fovea. Liquification of the vitreous is frequently found among those being treated for glaucoma with a miotic drug, such as pilocarpine. Iris nodules and other adverse symptoms also appear, not to mention the severe impairment of night vision by direct effects upon retinal sensitivity and by the extreme reduction of retinal illumination due to a small pupil.

FUNDUS STUDY

The fundus of the eye offers clues to retinal health as well as neurological and systemic health. Retinopathies or other evidences of active ocular pathology must be referred for medical attention. Visual symptoms would be reduced acuity, reduced contrast sensitivity, excessive vitreous floaters, poor night vision, distorted retinal images, and so on. Patients with evidences of untreated hypertension, arterio- or atherosclerosis, or diabetes should be referred for medical attention. A driver's license should not be permitted until cleared by a physician who is cognizant of the hazards of modern-day driving and the probable risk involved of a cardiac crisis occurring during driving. Patients showing physical signs of liability to episodes that could render them incapable of operating a motor vehicle should be told of the seriousness of attempting to drive. Notification should be sent to the driver licensing agency if the physical or ocular conditions noted seem to contraindicate safe driving.

INTRAOCULAR PRESSURE MEASUREMENTS

Intraocular pressure must be measured on all patients where symptoms or signs of glaucoma exist and on all patients forty years of age or older. Early glaucoma is not a basis for restricting driving day or night, provided the patient is not being treated with pilocarpine or some other miotic. However, when visual fields fall below the limit of 70 degrees to either side of the line of sight, the person usually should not be allowed to drive. Acute attacks of glaucoma cause increased ocular scatter similar to that seen through a lycopodium-powdered plate * and will definitely be a hazard to attempted night or even daytime driving. In addition the headache and nausea that often accompany acute glaucoma attacks would probably discourage a person from continuing to drive.

PHOTOMYOCLONIC, PHOTOCONVULSIVE, AND PHOTOPHOBIC TENDENCIES

High-intensity light flashes at 15 to 18 cycles per second produce widespread abnormal central nervous system responses in a few especially sensitive people (Allen and Courtney, 1967). It is believed that 1 out of about 250 epileptic patients will have a tendency to grand mal or petit mal epilepsy when exposed to a strong natural photic environment such as picket fences, dashed highway stripes, or tree shadows, viewed while moving in an automobile or while walking. Helicopters are especially hazardous to the pilot with photoconvulsive tendencies. Usually the patient has no prodromal warning, loses consciousness, and falls. The attacks last from a few minutes to twenty minutes or longer.

If the case history reveals any unexplained episodes of unconsciousness or other suspicious signs, patients who drive or whose occupations are potentially hazardous to themselves or others should be tested (Bickford 1948). A bright light viewed through a sectored disc chopping the light about 9 to 18 times per second should induce symptoms of an attack. Prodromal signs are a twitching of the eyelids and an interference in speech. In stroboscopic light the lid twitching might be noted only by palpation. It may take less than ten seconds to induce an attack. Ask the patient to count as long as he can while he faces the flickering light. If he falters he may be nearing unconsciousness. The Translid Binocular Interaction Trainer provides stimulation rates alternately to the eyes at 8 to 10 cycles per second. The Fusionaider gives 10 cycles per second alternately or simultaneously and should be used to chop the light from a 150-watt reflector flood lamp that is illuminating the closed eyelids from a distance of one to two feet. Resistance to either of these instruments for two to three minutes of exposure probably is adequate proof of freedom from photoconvulsive tendencies.

For therapy, treatments may be given consisting of photic driving while monitoring brain waves. Upon the first signs of epileptoform brain waves, the flashing light is turned off. When the brain rhythms have returned to normal, the flashing stimulus is again applied. Tolerance to flashing lights is thus built up in a few training periods. Without electroencephalographic equipment the same effects could probably be obtained by a cautious treatment program starting with one to five seconds of low-intensity light stimulation at 9 to 18 cycles per second followed by

---

* Made by dusting lycopodium powder over a clean plate of glass bearing a thin film of petroleum jelly and covering with a clean coverglass. Lycopodium powder is commonly available from a pharmacist.

thirty to sixty seconds of no stimulation. An increase should be made in the length of time of stimulation or in the intensity of the flashing light at each succeeding visit. When the patient can withstand several minutes of high-intensity flickering light, his resistance is probably beginning to be safe for driving.

There is also some evidence that red-free light will not cause photo convulsions. There are cases in the literature of epileptics, uncontrolled by drugs, becoming symptom free after wearing red-free filter glasses. The use of green lenses may also have merit in some of these cases and should be tried. The hazard, of course, is the insensitivity to red traffic signal lights while wearing red-free or green lenses. Such a person should not drive either with or without the colored glasses.

REFRACTION

OBJECTIVE TESTS

The foundation stone in refraction is retinoscopy. For improved reflex brightness and a larger patient pupil, a blue-free filter such as Corning's No. 3–67, glass No. 3482, could be placed over the retinoscope source. The older patient with excessive scattering in his eye, particularly in the blue end, will be easier to scope with the recommended filter. There should be less than an 0.25-diopter difference between the scope findings with and without the recommended filter.

A second item of importance to accurate retinoscopy is a spectacle made especially for the older optometrist to wear during retinoscopy. These spectacles should contain in the major portion of the lens the examiner's distance prescription plus the value of the usual working-distance lens. A conventional near add will be needed for writing. Such a bifocal prescription provides an unobstructed view of the phoropter and an *in-focus* view of the *patient's pupil* through the uppers. The examiner must look at the reflex in the plane of the patient's pupil for accurate retinoscopy. This retinoscopy spectacle will improve accuracy, and make the reflex easier to see.

If the pupil size is small, retinoscopy cannot be done accurately at the usual distance. By scoping at 33 or 25 cm. and by wearing the correct retinoscopy lenses as a fit over to allow a clear view of the patient's pupil, the difficulties of scoping a small pupil may be circumvented. However, since ophthalmoscopy also is difficult with a small pupil, it is wise in such cases to dilate the pupils, using one or two drops of 10 percent ophthalmic Neo-synephrine in each eye. Dilation should begin to occur within twenty minutes and be complete in thirty minutes. The effects should wear off in two to four hours. Visual fields should be taken as well as ophthalmoscopy and retinoscopy while the pupils are dilated.

This will give a truer measure of field defects and hence of retinal health. However, for a driver's visual field test, the pupils should be at their normal size.

Another objective test, keratometry, can reveal evidences of elevated intraocular pressure because the cornea becomes irregular or bumpy at elevated pressures. This will cause the mires to look distorted or irregular and may cause corneal power readings to be different from time to time. A hazy corneal stroma or an irregular corneal surface precludes good visual acuity and suggests glaucoma.

SUBJECTIVE TESTS

MONOCULAR. A patient with a small pupil cannot easily make the clarity judgments asked of him because of a large depth of focus and because of a reduced light level at the retina. Dilation of the pupil with 10 percent Neo-synephrine is helpful just as it is in retinoscopy. Raising light levels on the test screen and on the walls of the refracting room will also help. The refraction might be done with a cardboard wall chart and about 250 watts of reflector flood lighting placed about two and a half feet away from the chart instead of the regular projector test chart. It should be apparent to doctor and patient that night driving should be discouraged.

The red-green test is a generally useful test that requires some care. The filters are subject to fading, which reduces the sensitivity of the test: the red tends to become orange and the green tends to become yellow-green. In addition many filters, even when new, are not properly balanced both as to wavelength and total transmission. If the filters are a bright blue-green and a bright orange-red of equal intensity with the blue-green, you can be assured of good performance on the test. The red should actually appear brighter to a normal person, so that it will help the protanopic and protanomalous color defectives who are much less sensitive to red light. High-screen brightness will reduce the adverse effects of protanopia and of the small pupils and greater media absorption in the older patient.

For the red-green test the aluminized screen must appear dark when the projector is off, though the room should have 2 to 15 foot-candles of illumination on the walls. The aluminized screen should reflect like a mirror, directly toward the patient. The projector lenses and targets should be clean and aligned to provide a high-screen illumination. A higher wattage bulb in the projector will be beneficial. Caution: Some projectors cannot keep a high-wattage bulb cool, and the optics may be damaged by heat. A change from 50 to 100 watts is a safe change and will give more than a two-fold increase in screen luminance. Higher screen luminances as seen by the patient will speed up a subjective refraction and make it more accurate.

The fan dial test for astigmatism should be conducted under the right amount of blur, that is, the least amount to ensure control of the test. If a three-line pattern and progressively more blur is used, the patient will first see three out-of-focus lines, then two clear lines, then multiple clear fine lines, and finally only a uniform gray area; see Figure 5-2. Hence, upon asking which lines are clearest, one must also ask how many lines the patient sees. It is possible for the patient to pick out as clearest a pattern of two lines produced by blur circle interaction 90 degrees away instead of correctly choosing the less blurred three-line pattern which does not appear to be as clear. If a single-line pattern is used in the sunburst or clock dial, then often two clear lines are seen instead of a blurred single line.

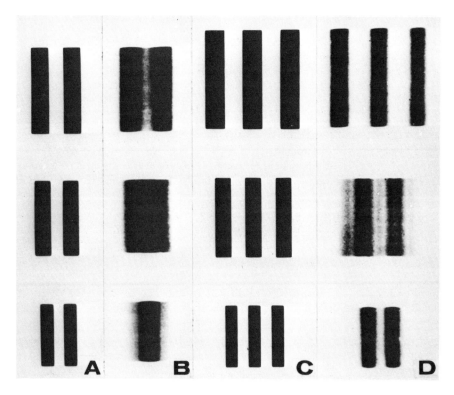

Figure 5-2. The effect of a given amount of cylindrical out-of-focus blur upon the image of two- and three-line targets of different sizes. This is equivalent to the image of the same target suffering different degrees of blur. Note that the two lines in A may appear as a single line in B, and three lines in C may appear as two in D when the blur is right. More intricate effects may occur in patients' eyes because the blur circle image for a point object is far more complex than the blur circle in the camera that took these photographs.

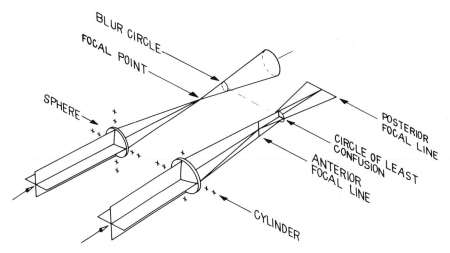

Figure 5-3. The diagram on the left represents the focusing of a bundle of light rays by a spherical lens. If the rays intercept a surface such as the retina at the position labeled BLUR CIRCLE, the light will be distributed in the circular area shown. In the diagram on the right the bundle of light rays is refracted by a cylindrical lens to produce an astigmatic focus. There is a position between the two focal lines which is called the CIRCLE OF LEAST CONFUSION and resembles the spherical blur circle in the left diagram. The crossed cylinder test, properly applied, alternately increases and reduces the distance between the two focal lines and thus makes the Circle of Least Confusion larger or smaller. This gives the patient an easy choice of which position of the crossed cylinder gives the clearest focus (smallest Blur Circle). People with astigmatism see things blurred but not slanted, as popularly depicted. The slant or distortion occurs when spectacles are used to correct the astigmatism. Contact lenses produce virtually no distortion.

Similarly, locating the middle of the astigmatic interval upon the retina (see Figure 5-3) is critical to the success of the Jackson cross cylinder test. The standard procedure is to add +0.25 diopter sphere for every −0.50 diopter of cylinder to keep the proper condition of "no blur." If the patient keeps rejecting minus cylinder in the crossed cylinder test for cylinder power, add an 0.25-diopter plus sphere and retest. If he keeps asking for more minus cylinder, give an 0.25-diopter minus sphere. Usually this is enough to reverse the patient's pattern of answers and to bring them back into agreement with the objectively determined cylinder.

BINOCULAR. If a patient's acuity is good in each eye, if his pupils are equal, and if he is binocular, the blur balance test is acceptable. If acuities are not the same, then a balance by blurring should not be used. A good test is the red-green used binocularly with vertical dissociation. If acuities are too poor for this test (20/40 or poorer), the retinoscope finding or the monocular subjective maximum plus sphere should be used to establish the balance.

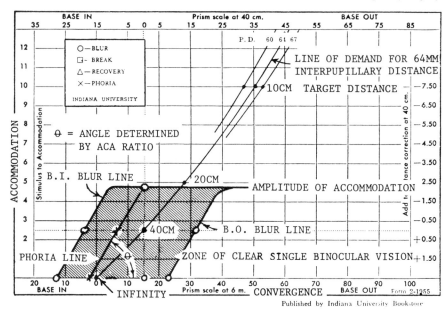

Figure 5-4. The zone of clear single binocular vision is indicated by the cross-hatched area. The hypothetical patient whose data are diagrammed here has a 2 exophoria, a base-out blur of 23 prism diopters, and a base-in blur of 13 prism diopters all at distance (infinity). At 40 centimeters, he has 8 exophoria, a base-out blur of 16 prism diopters, a base-in blur of 19 prism diopters, a plus lens to blur of +2.50 diopters, and a minus lens to blur of −2.25 diopters. His amplitude of accommodation is 4.75 diopters, and his A.C.A. ratio is about 3.33. The line of demand is curved because accommodation and convergence are not measured from a common point.

The Turville infinity balance test is excellent as a means of determining the subjective and for checking aniseikonia, vertical phoria, and lateral phoria tendencies. When using a direct view of a projected test target, the septum in the middle of the room should be fixed while the projected image on the screen is shifted about to get the proper left- and right-eye view. Polarizing techniques are available and the principles of testing are much the same. Though polarizing techniques simplify alignment, a serious light loss occurs which interferes with its use for older patients unless luminances are increased per the discussion in the section on Monocular Subjective Tests.

An effective "binocular" test may be performed with both eyes open but with one blurred by about +1.00 diopter. The best subjective refraction of the clearer eye is determined; then the one diopter blur is moved from one eye to the other, and the best refraction of the second eye is determined.

FIVE FUNDAMENTAL VARIABLES
OF OCULAR MUSCLE COORDINATION

1. DISTANCE PHORIA

The phoria at distance is the position of rest of the lines of sight of the two eyes in the absence of fusional and accommodative innervation. The classical distance phoria provides the starting point in building an understanding of the five important interrelationships between accommodation and convergence. Using the phoria as a starting position, the amount of fusional innervation needed for a given target will be proportional to the amount and direction of the distance phoria from ortho. The distance phoria in turn is somewhat affected by the direction, duration, and amount of fusional innervation as well as upon classical considerations such as orbital fat, extraocular muscle size and strength, check ligaments, and orbital shape.

The test for a distance phoria involves zero stimulus to accommodation and no fusion stimulus. If a large distance phoria exists or an intermittent tropia is present, the patient should be warned of hazards in driving late at night where the conditions approach a phoria test; that is, no stimulus to accommodation or to fusion. In many squinters it is typical that the ability to maintain single vision depends upon keeping the eyes at their normal squint angle. Night driving removes many of the important visual orientation clues, and hence a squinter cannot be relied upon to remain fully compensated at night or in fog.

2. POSITIVE FUSIONAL CONVERGENCE

The ability to increase convergence from the phoria position without increasing accommodation is called *positive fusional convergence*. It is of importance when an exophoria (out-turning tendency) exists, for it is the chief means of compensating for an exophoria. It appears to be impossible to induce fusional convergence by any means other than with a binocular fusional stimulus. It is a relatively slow posture adjustment which is easier to induce gradually with variable power prisms than to induce suddenly with a quick change in prism. With the lids closed the eyes tend to revert to the phoria position. Upon opening the eyes, a double image is seen until a fusional movement has occurred. Recovery findings in the blur-break-recovery prism tests give some idea of the ability to recover fusion. For example, a high exophoria and a low positive fusional amplitude as measured with the base out prism to blur test indicates a need for a spectacle prescription and/or visual therapy and advice to avoid night driving until the condition is corrected.

3. Negative Fusional Convergence

The ability to decrease convergence from the phoria position without a change in accommodation is called *negative fusional convergence*. Negative fusional convergence is the opposite of positive fusional convergence and becomes important in visual analysis when an esophoria (tendency to turn inward) exists. A weak negative fusional convergence ability or a high esophoria or both indicates a susceptibility to seeing double under adverse conditions, because most adverse conditions, such as blur, fog, darkness, fatigue, or alcohol, tend to increase the esophoria. Visual therapy and/or abstinence from night driving are indicated.

4. Amplitude of Accommodation

The accommodative amplitude is an indication of the flexibility of seeing clearly at all distances. The amplitude limits the near approach of an object to be seen clearly. The lower the amplitude, the longer it takes to change accommodation and the more difficult it is to see objects nearby, such as the instrument panel. In some ways a reduced amplitude is favorable for driving because it precludes accommodative spasms which may occur in an empty field, at low levels of illumination (night myopia), and after drinking alcohol or exposure to hypoxia or carbon monoxide. Multifocals for dash panel and map reading are essential for safe driving when a low amplitude is present.

5. A.C.A. Ratio

The letters A.C.A. stand for *accommodative convergence accommodation*. The A.C.A. ratio is defined as the amount of convergence change induced by an accommodative change of 1 diopter. We know a great deal about the A.C.A. ratio, but we do not know how to make permanent changes in it. Pathological or pharmaceutical attacks on the accommodative mechanism can cause the A.C.A. ratio to rise. Impairments of the convergence mechanism will cause it to fall. Many factors are contributory, such as the strength and attachment of the medial recti muscles, the ciliary muscle size, and the zonular fiber strength and arrangement. Even so, the A.C.A. ratio is surprisingly constant for a given individual month after month.

Whatever the causative factors, an A.C.A. ratio outside the limits of 4/1 to 6/1 is abnormal and can contribute to discomfort in reading and driving and even contribute to diplopia and confusion under certain conditions. If the abnormal A.C.A. is of a transient nature, as for example a high A.C.A. ratio resulting from atropine in medications for colds or ulcers, it is only necessary to wait a few weeks after cessation of medication for it to return to normal. If the abnormal A.C.A. ratio is a "natural"

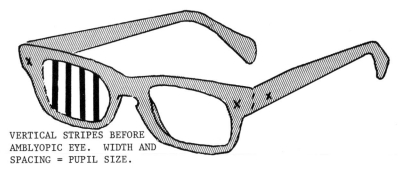

VERTICAL STRIPES BEFORE
AMBLYOPIC EYE. WIDTH AND
SPACING = PUPIL SIZE.

Figure 5-5. Vertical stripes applied to a spectacle lens provide a unique stimulus to an amblyopic eye or a means of increasing binocular interaction. No serious interference with the field of view occurs when such a partial occluder is worn in contrast with complete uniocular occlusion. (Adapted from Oppenheimer, 1968.)

condition for the patient, appropriate lens and/or prism corrections should be provided—usually as a multifocal. If a hazard of diplopia exists under low levels of illumination, visual therapy should be given to ensure that diplopia will not occur. Such therapy would include stress prisms or lenses, large excursion rotations, and eye-hand coordination training using a rotating pegboard and a training occluder (Oppenheimer, 1968) see Figure 5-5. Stress prisms would be base in for a high A.C.A. ratio and base out for a low A.C.A. ratio. Stress lenses would be minus for a high A.C.A. ratio; but for an A.C.A. ratio of less than 3/1, stress lenses are not appropriate.

SPECIAL TESTS

Aniseikonia

Aniseikonia is a difference in image size of the two eyes. It can be meridional or overall and can be a serious problem in spatial orientation. Aniseikonia is usually considered to be induced by spectacle differences or differences in the lengths of the two eyes. However, photo-receptor distribution and cortical representations from the two eyes are equally important factors in aniseikonia. Indeed—like refractive errors and phorias—the wonder is that there are so few people with a significant amount of aniseikonia of 5 percent or more.

Adaptation to a new pair of glasses is usually strangely distressing for a few minutes, hours, or days, but within two weeks it is usually complete. If a person has an appreciable natural aniseikonia, it is possible that his binocular abilities have never been fully developed and that a program of building normal binocular function will permit a successful adaptation to the aniseikonia. Heavy emphasis should be placed on the maintenance of binocular vision while spatial orientation training, such as baseball, table tennis, or rotating pegboard, is practiced.

In any event, aniseikonic spatial distortions, like chromestereopsis errors, usually show up only when normal perspective clues are missing or are unreliable. This occurs in the leaf room * or behind the wheel of an automobile late at night when other automobiles are seldom encountered and when fatigue has reduced the driver's compensating ability. The symptoms of aniseikonia then will be illusions of going up or down hills, or being on a roadway that slopes to the right or left, or suffering a combination of these effects. A sudden loss of normal perspective and overlay spatial clues could create a dangerous illusion for the aniseikonic patient when driving; this could result in disorientation, confusion, and perhaps an accident.

Aniseikonia is suspected when refractive and muscle balance corrections have been supplied and headaches or asthenopia persist. Further evidence is supplied if, after monocular occlusion for a few days, the symptoms do not occur. The aniseikonia would then have to be differentiated from cyclophoria, lateral phoria, or vertical phoria anomalies, which can cause the same symptom complex.

It is never safe to rely upon assumptions about aniseikonia based upon refractive considerations alone, except where a person of known good binocularity has been comfortable and we are contemplating a change in base curves or thickness, as in safety glasses or lenses after cataract surgery. Then we can use his present base curves, thicknesses, prescription powers, and vertex distances to determine intelligently these variables in the new prescription. Otherwise the only safe procedure is to measure the amount of aniseikonia with an Eikonometer through the new prescription and to redesign one or both lenses as needed to bring the Eikonometer reading to zero.

Eikonometry can only be done if normal binocular vision with stereopsis is present. Binocular anomalies of suppression, anomalous correspondence, amblyopia, and strabismus can result from aniseikonia. But persons with such anomalies cannot be tested with an Eikonometer because they do not have stereopsis. A technique based upon afterimages has been recommended by William Ludlam, O.D., of the Optometric Center of New York. Put a pair of bright lines on a wall such as formed by a U-shaped high-intensity flash tube or a pair of parallel showcase bulbs. Induce an afterimage in the nonamblyopic eye. Occlude this eye

---

* The leaf room is a test room whose square corners and flat surfaces have been covered over with leaves hanging by their stems so that the normal appearance of the room is obliterated. Under such conditions, space distortions often become apparent, because the subject does not know what the room is supposed to look like.

and, using the other eye, have the patient walk toward or away from the wall until the afterimages in the occluded eye appear to be the same size as the pair of nonilluminated lines. The ratio of the distance used to induce the afterimage to the distance needed to make the second eye image the same size as the afterimage in the first eye is the measure of aniseikonia in the meridian measured. The shorter distance is used instead of a magnifying lens to equate the images. Keep in mind that at ten feet a one-foot difference between the viewing distances of the two eyes gives about a 10 percent size difference; hence distances must be carefully measured and the test repeated on several different office visits if any question of accuracy exists.

The formula for computing the magnifying effect (M) of a spectacle lens is as follows: M = shape magnification x power magnification.

$$M = \left(\frac{1}{1 - \frac{t}{n} F_1}\right) \times \left(\frac{1}{1 - aF'_v}\right)$$

Where F_1 = Front surface power

t = Center thickness of the lens

a = Distance of entrance pupil from back vertex of lens

F'_v = Back vertex power of the lens

The ratio of the magnification of each spectacle lens should be the same as the aniseikonia ratio to be corrected but opposite in sign; that is, the larger-imaged eye would need the smaller spectacle magnification.

Color Vision

Dalton in 1798 wrote about his own color vision defect as follows:

I found that persons in general distinguish six kinds of colour in the solar image, namely red, orange, yellow, green, blue, and purple. Newton, indeed, divides the purple into indigo and violet; but the difference between him and others is merely nominal. To me it is quite otherwise. I see only two, or at most three distinctions. These I should call yellow and blue, or yellow, blue and purple. My yellow comprehends the red, orange, yellow and green of others; my blue and purple coincide with theirs (Judd, 1943).

This lucid description of a visual problem clearly indicates the futility of designing a traffic-control signal system based upon color, as we now have, unless such defective drivers are an insignificant minority. The chief characteristic of color blindness is confusion of colors as compared to the normal observer, and about 8 percent of the male population has a permanent color vision defect of some sort. Very few females in comparison are so affected. Acquired color vision defects from injury or disease are also possible.

For all practical purposes color-defective people tend to confuse red, green, and yellow signals, but the color vision defect may be slight or severe. The tests of interest in diagnosing the several types of color vision defects follow.

The anomaloscope is an instrument for mixing red and green to match a yellow. The yellow is adjustable in brightness. An extra amount of red in the match indicates protanopia; of green, deuteranopia; and the ability to match any color combination of red plus green with yellow indicates absolute color blindness. Protanomaly and deuteranomaly are less severe degrees of protanopia and deuteranopia. The Nagel Anomaloscope * is the best known example of such instruments. The excellence of an anomaloscope depends upon how good the filters are, or what portions of the spectrum are used for matching, and how precisely measurements can be made of the proportions of colors and luminances needed to make the yellow and red plus green areas appear equal.

The Farnsworth 100 Hue Test ** consists of eighty-five plastic caps containing a series of graded Munsell papers that the patient arranges in a look-alike or matching-of-similar-colors sequence. Errors in placing the colors in proper order give clues to the anomaly.

The Farnsworth Dichomatous Test † is less time-consuming than the 100 Hue Test because it has only fifteen caps that must be arranged in a sequence of similar colors. It gives clear-cut indication in most cases of the type of defect present.

The American Optical Company Hardy, Rand, and Rittler ‡ (A.O.H.R.R.) Pseudoisochromatic test plates are perhaps the best of the book tests for color vision defects. Some indication of the type of defect can be obtained from this test, but in general this and other book tests such as the Dvorine, Ishihara are primarily intended as pass-fail tests.

In all tests one must maintain rigorous adherence to brightness levels and the quality of light used to illuminate the test colors. The recommended lamp source should be used at the prescribed distance if meaningful results are to be obtained. Color vision defects should be noted and the patient warned of the hazards in driving. Color defectives take longer to make decisions and make many errors compared to normal-sighted persons. If the optometrist is called upon to evaluate a person's ability to drive in the face of a color vision defect, a driving test is perhaps the only way to evaluate the ability of such a person to use the other factors that contribute information and make driving relatively safe in spite of color vision defects. Even so, night driving for color defectives might need

* Distributed in U.S. by Alfred P. Poll, 40 West 55th Street, New York, N.Y., 10019. A similar instrument has been manufactured by Bausch and Lomb Optical Company, Ophthalmic Division, 635 St. Paul Street, Rochester, N.Y., 14602.
** Munsell Color Corporation Inc., 2441 North Calvert Street, Baltimore, Md., 21218.
† The Psychological Corporation, 304 East 45th Street, New York, N.Y., 10017.
‡ The American Optical Company, Instrument Division, Buffalo, N.Y., 14215.

to be restricted to well-lighted streets and freeways. A protanope or protanomalous color defective will be very insensitive to red light and will be handicapped as he approaches an unfamiliar intersection or an obstacle showing only a red light.

The color defective can be helped to analyze a light by putting a small spot of red filter material on his glasses in the upper outer corner. If the light from an unidentified color passes through the red filter, he will know it is not green or blue and hence must be yellow, orange, or red.

STEREOPSIS

Stereopsis is the three-dimensional depth sense mediated through the simultaneous use of two eyes. Stereopsis gives relative perception of distance of one object compared to another. Perspective and overlay clues are also very important spatial clues which work quite well for people with one eye. Beyond about 3,000 feet stereopsis is not helpful in judging which object is nearer or farther away because of the small separation of the two eyes and the stereo-acuity limit of about 12 seconds of arc. In fact one would expect that objects at infinity would be just noticeably farther away than objects at 3,000 feet. In the event of a stereopsis illusion such as caused by chromatic aberration and a displaced pupil, lights of different color may be seen to be displaced in front of or behind their true position.

Stereopsis is highly desirable for maneuvering a school bus, tractor trailer, or automobile in parking, loading, or driving in closely spaced traffic. The absence of stereopsis means that a driver must obtain his spatial clues by perspective, overlay, relative intensity, and monocular parallax by weaving and bobbing his head. Like color vision, a lack of stereopsis may be evaluated as to its interference with safe driving by a performance test in the vehicle under realistic or actual operating conditions. Stereopsis for high-speed highway travel probably is not needed very much because viewing distances are usually great.

Stereopsis testing can be carried out with the classical peg test operated from twenty feet by the patient holding a string to bring a movable peg into side-by-side relationship with a fixed peg. The clever ways in which air cadets have defeated this test are legend. It is argued that stereopsis is an all-or-none phenomenon and that, if you have stereopsis, its excellence depends upon such factors as the accuracy of the binocular vision correction. On this basis a simple test like the stereo fly or the diastereo test (Hofstetter, 1968) is ample (see Figure 5-6). The latter is a flashlight with a frosted plastic face bearing three spots, one of which is elevated toward the observer. The test criterion may be a simple four correct out of six different presentations at different positions, since, by guessing, one would expect only two out of six correct answers. Hofstetter's studies indicate that those who failed this test, though otherwise nor-

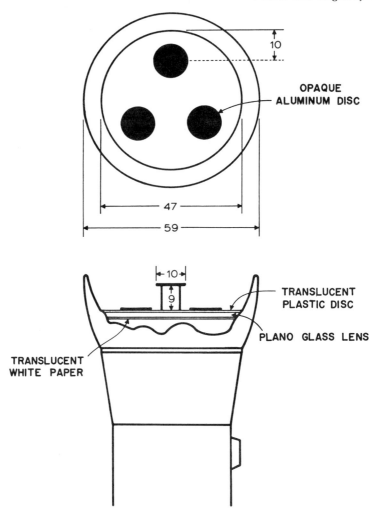

Figure 5-6. Cut-away showing the diastereo test flashlight (the dimensions given are in millimeters). The top view is that seen by the subject, who must select the black spot that appears nearest. A criterion of at least three correct responses out of four presentations at different positions seems adequate to eliminate the chance guess factor, which could give a passing score in the absence of stereopsis.

mal in superficial appearance, later turned out to be squinters who had been overlooked in a routine clinic examination.

Night Visual Performance

Driving performance at night may be significantly handicapped by the lack of light. This impairment comes about because of the following factors: (a) Reduction in illumination levels at night reduces the visual information available to the driver. (b) Lowered retinal illumination permits pupil dilation, which increases the optical aberrations and reduces the depth of focus. (c) Visual acuity falls with lowered light levels so that 20/20 by day will be considerably poorer under night seeing conditions. Acuity deteriorates more with some observers than with others, depending upon the condition of their eyes. (d) Brightness contrast sensitivity is reduced at low levels of illumination; hence easily seen objects of 5 percent contrast at room lighting levels become invisible at roadway illumination levels. (e) Photochemical dark adaptation makes seeing possible at the low levels of night driving. This process is adversely affected by pre-exposure to bright light even up to twelve or more hours beforehand. Hence it is desirable to protect the driver's eyes from excessive daylight if good performance is desired at night. (f) High altitudes provide lowered oxygen partial pressures in the atmosphere, lowered oxygen tension at the individual body cell, and impaired dark adaptation. Dark adaptation test

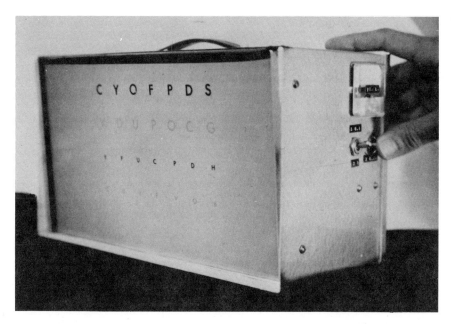

Figure 5-7. The Night Vision Performance Tester. This is one of several models of a device which provides low-contrast test letters against a background of variable luminance. By choosing a large illuminated area around the test letters, the influence of room illumination is reduced. By increasing the background luminance from zero, a level is reached where high-contrast letters will be readable. More background luminance is needed to read letters of lowered contrast. Similarly, when the eye reduces the retinal image contrast by blur or stray light, more light will be required. If the pupil is small or if an excess light absorption occurs in the ocular media, more light will be required also. Low-contrast test letters make the test more sensitive to ocular scatter and transmission losses.

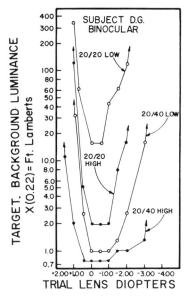

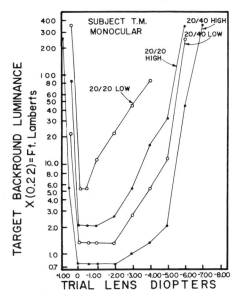

Figure 5-8. The effect of simulated myopia (+ lenses) and simulated hyperopia (− lenses) upon the night vision performance tester background luminance for a twenty-year-old binocular subject reading 20/20 and 20/40 high and low contrast letters.

Figure 5-9. The effect of simulated myopia (+ lenses) and simulated hyperopia (− lenses) upon the night vision performance tester background luminance for a forty-year-old subject tested monocularly. Figures 5-8 and 5-9 show the dependence of acuity upon contrast and luminance levels as classically shown in Figure 9-2 A and B. In addition, the devastating effect upon visual performance of blur due to refractive errors is shown as a need for more light.

performance is adversely affected by vitamin A deficiency, a small pupil, absorption and scatter in the crystalline lens, and the refractive error.

Since night driving requires many facets of vision besides the absolute light sensitivity threshold called scotopic vision and since nighttime driving is done at mesopic and low photopic levels rather than at the scotopic levels with which dark adaptation testing is usually involved, a performance test at the levels of night driving, or a predictor of performance at such levels, is needed.

The Night Vision Performance Tester is one such test for predicting night vision performance. Figure 5-7 shows the details of this apparatus, which in essence is a low-contrast 20/40 test letter viewed against a background of variable luminance and protected from room illumination by a layer of filters. The normally encountered room reflections from the filter surfaces are eliminated by angling the filters so that they reflect only from a black surface. Two instruments using this principle have been designed. One has a large luminance range and is suitable for office use in measuring age deterioration effects upon vision and in measuring subtle improvements in vision performance due to refractive refinements, diet, or medical treatments. The second instrument is a pass-fail instrument with brightness adjustability sufficient only to compensate for source aging. Both instruments contain photosensitive equipment for ensuring specified brightness levels.

Figures 5-8 and 5-9 show the deterioration of visual performance when tested with the Night Vision Performance Tester using lenses to simulate ametropia. Figure 5-10 shows the effect of refractive error upon nighttime visual performance in detecting a black or white obstacle the size of an automobile. Figure 5-11 shows the effect of wearing filters upon the test scores.

The Night Vision Performance Tester yields a score in terms of the illumination needed to see a given target; hence it provides a real indication of the light levels that will be needed for nighttime driving. The tester measures overall visual performance whatever the factors; these factors are pupil size, ocular transmission, ocular scatter, retinal pathologies, physiological abnormalities, and refractive errors.

The American Automobile Association Glareometer contains a pair of lights simulating headlights and a series of target patterns to be identified. The lower the illumination level on the targets needed to recognize them, the better the performance on the test.

The Porto Glare test exposes the subject to a bright headlight glare source. The time needed to recognize a test object after being exposed to this glare is a measure of glare recovery ability.

None of the above three tests has been evaluated against the actual driving performance of drivers at night, and hence it is not known whether one is superior to another. It is conceivable that they are measuring different things and that one may correlate better with driving performance than another. On a theoretical basis one might consider that all measure different aspects of the same thing and that they are thus more or less equivalent. From the optometric standpoint, however, the Night Vision Performance Tester is useful for other purposes as well; hence it would seem to be the choice for office use.

VISUAL FIELDS

All patients, young or old, should have a visual fields check at each eye examination. There is a good correlation between visual field defects and poor health, and the mapping of a visual field is analogous to the neurologist mapping the pain- and temperature-sensitive areas on the skin and studying sensory-motor reflexes. Such information permits the expert to pinpoint the location and the probable kind of lesion affecting the nerve pathways. With visual field mapping and checking for other

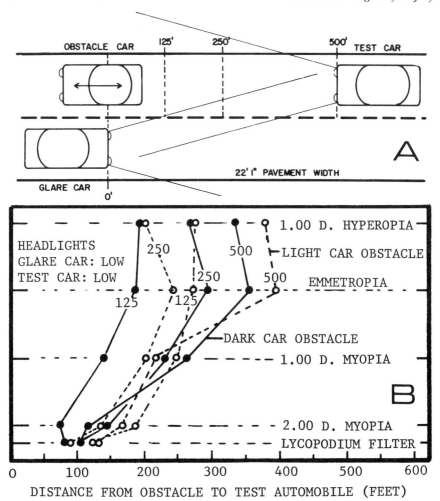

Figure 5-10. Part A shows the experimental arrangement of vehicles used to gather the data in part B. The rear of the obstacle car faced the observer in the test car. A white compact car covered with a white cloth was the light car obstacle. A black compact car covered with a black cloth was the dark car obstacle. The test car was placed at 125, 250, and 500 feet from the glare car. The obstacle car was moved toward the test car until detected. Part B shows that myopia and simulated glaucoma and cataract (lycopodium filter) caused startling losses in the detection distance of an obstacle as large as an automobile. Even the presence of hyperopia reduced performance somewhat in this twenty-six-year-old subject.

neurological symptoms, brain tumors, abscesses, aneurysms, infarcts, and hemorrhages can be located or ocular pathology revealed. Because visual fields testing is so easy, few realize its tremendous practical value. For example, if "Glaucoma Day" screening efforts were centered around a tangent screen instead of a tonometer, the yield would include nearly three times more *actual* glaucoma victims than are now detected; and, in addition, brain tumors, retinopathies, cataracts, and such blinding systemic diseases as diabetes would be detected. Another bonus would be a drop in the *over-referral* rate for glaucoma from such screening.

Nowadays it is no longer necessary to remain with the tangent screen, which for all its simplicity is as accurate as anyone might care to make it. The multiple pattern screener type of instrument offers a fast, reasonably efficient means of screening the major portions of the central visual fields. Studies have indicated that any peripheral vision defect will show up in some way as a central field anomaly in about 98 percent of the cases. It is justifiable therefore to perform the multiple pattern screener test on every optometric patient, and if the patient does poorly he should be studied in detail with a tangent screen. Since the eye changes with age, when using the multiple pattern screener for older observers adjust the room light downward until some spots can be seen fairly easily upon flash presentations. If the patient then detects all spots in all positions presented, he has no field defect. A younger observer would find that the lowered room illumination of the older man would make the test too easy, and the room light should be brightened until he is near the threshold for seeing the dots.

Projection self-recording tangent screens, projection photographic recording screens, and pantographic self-recording screens are now available to simplify and speed the tangent screen test.

Driver licensing requirements, usually set at 140 degrees of visual field, give a generous margin for inattention and tester ineptness, but if a visual field is actually reduced to this amount, the patient is surely in need of medical or optometric help. Optometric examination can establish the amount of the field defect and its significance for possible referral and the possible need to stop driving.

REACTION TIME

A reaction time test gives information on the total performance potential of an individual. If a sharp, bright retinal image is received and if the neurological components between the eye and the responding skeletal muscles are operating at optimum efficiency, the patient will have a fast reaction time. On the other hand, a blurred, low-contrast, low-intensity retinal image reduces the strength of the input signal and the reaction time will be longer. Similarly alcohol, drugs, fatigue, and cortical ischemia due to arterio- or atherosclerosis will cause a longer reaction time. If in addition there is neurological damage or loss of tissue, the reaction time will be further lengthened. Normal young active people have simple visual reaction times between 0.18 and 0.20 second. If a sound signal is present, the reaction time may become primarily auditory and speed up to 0.15 second. In experimental situations on the highway, visual reaction times from signal change to brake application exceed 0.5 second. In normal highway traffic a reaction time of 2.5 seconds upward may be expected.

Since the reaction time cuts across so many functional systems and gives a measure of performance which can reflect on driving ability, it seems reasonable that licensing agencies should begin testing visual reaction times. Police on accident investigation might well measure driver reaction times as well as blood alcohol levels. It is a simple test, and it will undoubtedly rise to a position of importance in license bureau testing and in optometric offices.

GLAUCOMA

Optometric testing for glaucoma should include the case history, the optometric examination, the use of some test for visual field integrity, and the use of a tonometer. Reputable authorities classify chronic simple glaucoma as a symptom and not a disease in its own right. Authorities also agree that it is not clear whether increased intraocular pressure causes the visual field defects or whether the process causing the field defects also causes the elevated pressures which are often, but not always, observed.

Since so little agreement exists on the association of a markedly elevated pressure in the eye with peripheral vision loss, it is essential that a glaucoma detection procedure or a blindness prevention program rely upon the case history, fundus examination, central vision, and visual field studies as important prognosticators of health. The tonometer must be used also, for it may indicate an abnormality unnoted by any of the other procedures.

The presence of glaucoma presupposes visual field defects, either partial or absolute, which would make driving hazardous; the more so, the larger the defect. Glaucoma—using the word to mean *elevated pressure* —is associated with increased intraocular scatter of light, mostly from the cornea. Stressing the cornea causes a distortion of corneal stroma fibrils which reduces corneal transparency by increasing the amount of scattered light. The increase in scatter is reported to be proportional to the increase in pressure within the eye; hence a slit lamp or ophthalmoscopic impression of increased corneal scatter should suggest increased intraocular pressure. Except in an active inflammatory process (or residual clouding from an old one,) almost no other cause for increased corneal clouding is commonly encountered. When the pressure reverts to normal ranges, the clouding subsides unless there has been a permanent disruption of stromal fibers.

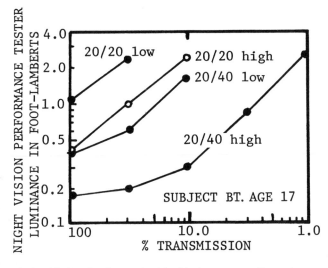

Figure 5-11. The effect of a reduced ocular transmission with age is simulated with neutral density filters before the eyes of a seventeen - year - old subject. One possible reason that a straight-line relationship was not obtained is that the pupil tends to compensate for the lowered retinal luminance occurring with the filters. Increased ocular absorption should thus be detected with this instrument. Since about twice as much light is needed to perform the same visual task for each thirteen-year increase in age, a lifetime can cause a need for over 50 times more light compared to a thirteen-year-old. Yet Figure 7-5 shows that the actual transmission change of the eye between a two-year-old and a seventy-five-year-old is not likely to exceed 2.5 times. Probably a degradation in optical image quality and retinal function and a change in pupil size accounts for the differences.

Glaucoma affects driving ability by causing visual field defects, by increased ocular scatter and by reduced night vision capability. The patient treated for glaucoma with pilocarpine has a small pupil which reduces retinal illumination to about 1/9, assuming a 2-mm. pilocarpine pupil compared to a 6-mm. pupil normally expected under night driving conditions. There is also some evidence that pilocarpine has an adverse effect upon the retina itself and thus further interferes with nighttime seeing. Certainly monocular treatment with pilocarpine is an undesirable procedure so far as it concerns fitness to drive by day or night. The monocular meiosis causes severe spatial distortions of the Pulfrich type, similar to wearing a filter over the miotic eye. The treatment of glaucoma by a sympathomimetic drug such as Neo-synephrine causes a large pupil, and thus there is no handicap for night driving. Combination drugs are available which keep a fairly normal pupil size. Diamox given by mouth will hold pressures in line for long periods, while glycerine given by mouth is useful in lowering intraocular pressure in a crisis. All such treatments are symptomatic. For a cure it appears that other health factors must be evaluated and improved as needed. For example, both improved nutrition and exercise have been shown to favorably affect intraocular pressure.

Chapter 6: Prescribing for Driving

DAYTIME DRIVING

LENS POWER

THE PROPER PRESCRIPTION for daytime driving has not been extensively studied; however, certain indications help us to make a rational decision. Outdoor people do not like to wear a full plus prescription, preferring to have up to 0.50 diopter of accommodation in play at distance. Indoor people, on the other hand, easily accept full plus at distance, apparently to obtain the relief of reduced strain on their accommodative mechanism at near.

Luckiesh et al (1940, 1941, 1943, 1949), using the Sensitometric Method of refraction, concluded that the best prescription at distance was up to 1.00 diopter less plus than normally prescribed. The phenomena of night myopia, empty field myopia, and blurred or fogged-vision myopia indicate exactly the same thing for prepresbyopes: namely, that accommodation of about 1.00 diopter is natural when no stimuli are present. Myopes tend to show less and uncorrected hyperopes to show more accommodative tonicity. The phenomenon of night myopia is somewhat different in that both spherical aberration, due to an enlarged pupil, and a shift in spectral sensitivity toward the blue end of the spectrum account for up to 1.00 diopter of the condition, which may exceed 1.50 diopters.

For the normal clinical determination of the best distance prescription for daytime driving the duochrome test is recommended as the test of choice. When testing binocularly in a twenty-foot room, leave the presbyopic patient slightly clearer on the green letter side. For the prepresbyope the amount to undercorrect at distance would be determined by the following considerations:

A patient with a high A.C.A. ratio will probably accept full plus up to the slight preference for green of the presbyope. An uncorrected hyperope receiving his first glasses will not accept the full plus. The less acceptance occurs with younger drivers and with the greater amount of previously uncorrected hyperopia. The uncorrected myope is likely to accept the maximum plus red-equals-green prescription without complaint, although a higher minus might give better vision. Strange as it may seem, the flexibility of accommodation demanded by the hyperope may actually be the cause of discomfort for many myopes. The best prescription may be either in spectacle lenses or contact lenses.

The correction of astigmatism should be complete so long as the axes are at or near the 90- or 180-degree meridian. The person with a high amount of astigmatism, over 1.50 diopters with oblique axes, will have both a significant spatial distortion problem and an anisophoria involving both vertical and horizontal components if spectacles are prescribed. While a full prescription is recommended for best visual acuity for all astigmatic errors, for oblique axis astigmatism the spectacle problems involved suggest that a better way might be to prescribe contact lenses.

SPECTACLE FRAMES

It is unfortunately true that at the same time that automotive vision experts extol the virtues of unlimited visibility without obstructions or distortions, the ophthalmic practitioners provide both obstructions and distortions in the eye wear they dispense (Bewley, 1969). Frames with heavy eye wires and bulky temples are commonplace. Visually superior frames and mountings are not recommended by the experts, who seem to prefer the easier approach of letting fashion dictate eye-wear styles. That these are poor choices is well known to everyone who dispenses and has to adjust, repair, straighten, or glaze many of the more popular styles.

Simply stated, a pair of lenses is a visual aid and should permit unrestricted vision throughout the visual field, both with the fovea and the peripheral retina. The edges of high plus lenses cause a blind zone which is a function of the power of the prescription, the diameter of the lens, and the distance from the eye. High minus lenses, on the other hand, even with thick edges, provide a field overlap and hence no blind area. To put the plus lens blind area as far in the periphery as possible requires large lenses of high base curve and a fit that is close to the eyes. Many wrap-around sunglasses achieve this effect reasonably well, but prescription lenses cannot usually be made this way.

The steeper the base curve, the less distortion produced by a spectacle lens. However, a minus-power corrected curve lens with good marginal performance is flatter as the minus power increases; hence distortion may become a problem even though edge-to-edge visual acuity may be quite good. By using globular lenses (Wollaston portion of the Tscherning ellipse) both astigmatism and distortion are minimized. This is a reasonable approach mechanically for low-power minus lenses, but for high powers the curves are not practical to manufacture by the laboratory; even if they were, the lenses would be of very small overall diame-

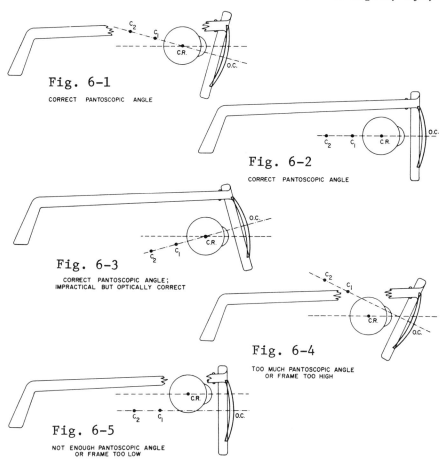

Fig. 6-1
CORRECT PANTOSCOPIC ANGLE

Fig. 6-2
CORRECT PANTOSCOPIC ANGLE

Fig. 6-3
CORRECT PANTOSCOPIC ANGLE;
IMPRACTICAL BUT OPTICALLY CORRECT

Fig. 6-4
TOO MUCH PANTOSCOPIC ANGLE
OR FRAME TOO HIGH

Fig. 6-5
NOT ENOUGH PANTOSCOPIC ANGLE
OR FRAME TOO LOW

Figures 6-1 through 6-5. Placement of spectacle lenses. Figures 6-1, 6-2, and 6-3 show optically correct placement, while Figures 6-4 and 6-5 are incorrect. Corrected curve lenses are designed for an eye whose center of rotation (C.R.) is located on the optic axis of the lens. The optic axis is the line joining C_2, C_1, and O.C. The pantoscopic or spectacle tilt angle is thus interrelated with the vertical position of the lenses before the eyes. Frames that do not maintain the desired lens placement thus impair the performance of the lens prescription, adding errors and distortions of their own.

ter. Hence to correct a high myope properly, because of distortions, the use of contact lenses is indicated; for high hyperopes and aphakics, the blind zone at the edge of the lens dictates contact lenses or very large spectacle lenses fitted as close to the eyes as feasible.

The proper spectacle frame is one that accurately and reliably places the lenses at their design distance and angle with an absolute minimum of obstruction in the field of view, with one important exception. Overhead lights and the open sky cause considerable distress and eyebrow lowering; hence spectacle frames that add to the shading effect of the eyebrows are beneficial. The use of nylon bands and/or thin metal for the eye wires provides an attractive, practical, nonobstructive spectacle frame. Temples that are high, at eyebrow level, and are not more than one quarter inch wide are acceptable.

After a pair of glasses has been placed on the patient's face the accuracy of the height and pantoscopic tilt must be checked to ensure optimum performance of the lenses. A retinoscope, ophthalmoscope, or penlight held close to the fitter's eye can be used as a source to show the optic axis of the lens and the line of sight of the patient's eye (Allen, April 1962). While the patient is fixating the source, the fitter moves around until the reflections from the two surfaces of the lens coincide. If they are also centered in the patient's pupil, the lens is properly aligned; see Figures 6-1 through 6-5. If the lens reflections and the center of the pupil do not coincide, tilting the lenses or raising or lowering them will correct the error. Sometimes it is neccessary to change the plane of the frame by bending it back or forward at the bridge to correct a lateral misalignment; see Figures 6-6 through 6-10.

If prism is present, optimum corrected-curve lens performance can be obtained if the optic axis passes through the sighting center (C.R.) of the eye as indicated in the figures, even though this means that the frame needs to be bent back at the bridge to angle the temporal edge of the lenses nearer to the face or vice versa. In any event the optic axes of the lenses need not be parallel for optimum corrected-curve performance on a given patient.

This problem is important in all cases where spectacles are used for vision correction, but it becomes extremely important when lens powers of 1.50 diopters and over are required. Failure to observe proper alignment causes distortion of familiar surroundings as well as a loss in acuity due to aberration powers (sphere and cylinder) which are not found in the lens when it is properly positioned. Greater attention to spectacle optics will improve the patient's acceptance of a new pair of glasses and should materially shorten the time needed to adapt to them. It will also reduce the complications of confusion and dizziness that spectacle distortions induce in dynamic situations such as driving.

SUNGLASSES

There are two kinds of data available on sunglasses. The one type evaluates the visual performance through the sunglass, while the other considers its protective aspects. A study of visual performance through sunglass filters was made by the author, using a high-intensity room under various degrees of clear and fog atmosphere. Fog was controlled at 0, 50, and 75 percent scattered light for room wall luminances of 470 to 7,000 foot-lamberts. The filters used were:

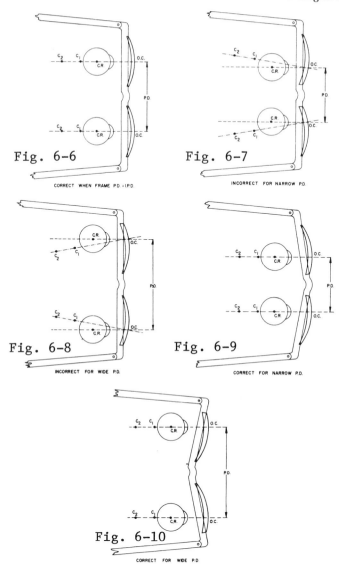

Fig. 6-6

CORRECT WHEN FRAME P.D. : I.P.D.

Fig. 6-7

INCORRECT FOR NARROW P.D.

Fig. 6-8

INCORRECT FOR WIDE P.D.

Fig. 6-9

CORRECT FOR NARROW P.D.

Fig. 6-10

CORRECT FOR WIDE P.D.

Figures 6-6 through 6-10. The relationship between patient interpupillary distance (P.D.) and the optical axes of the spectacle lenses. Figure 6-6 is the normal situation in which the optical center (O.C.) of the lenses and the patient's P.D. agree. Spectacle lenses are customarily aligned in the frame so the back surfaces lie in a plane as shown. Figures 6-7 and 6-8 show the complication of maintaining a flat spectacle plane when the patient's P.D. does not agree with the spectacle P.D. The lens O.C.s agree with the P.D., but the optical axes of the lenses do not pass through the C.R. of the patient's eyes as required for optimum lens performance. Figures 6-9 and 6-10 show the remedy that may be obtained by bending the plane of the frame at the center or by special edge treatment of the lenses so they are properly angled when inserted in a flat frame.

TABLE 6-1

Ophthalmic Filter	No Coating % Transmission	Uniform Coating % Transmission	Gradient Coating % Transmission		
			Top	Center	Bottom
White	100% (no lenses)	10.2%	1.5%	8.0%	91.5%
Azurelite	40%	10.0%	.6%	2.4%	38.7%
Calobar	25.8%	Defective coating	.2%	13.1%	24.7%
G-15	16.3%	Defective coating	.3%	14.0%	16.0%
Smoke Rose	21.8%	Defective coating	.2%	12.2%	22.2%
Kalichrome	81.0%	13.8%	1.0%	7.4%	73.0%

The uniform and gradient coatings were supplied by American Metal Lux (now a subsidiary of the American Optical Corporation). The coating material had uniform absorption for all wavelengths across the visible spectrum varying from 11 percent to 12.5 percent transmission on the sample tested. All filter-coated lenses were also antireflection coated, which reduced the mirrorlike reflections enough to resemble the reflections from ordinary glass. The coating was on the side nearest the eye and was kept free of oil and water, which would have caused an increase in surface reflections. Fifteen pairs of sunglasses, all in identical air force frames, were used on each of six subjects, who made threshold brightness measurements at twenty feet and reaction-time responses to a near target on the dash panel. Measurements were made of the time required to recognize the position of the gap in a Landolt C target presented at random and in either of two windows on an aircraft instrument panel.

The results at 400 foot-lamberts, which is about the average luminance under an overcast sky, showed that *no* sunglasses gave the best visual performance. At 7,000 foot-lamberts, which is about as bright as the sky ever gets except very near the sun, both the performance and comfort were improved with sunglasses. The darker sunglasses gave the better performances. The yellow (Kalichrome) sunglasses were especially disliked by all subjects when room intensities went above 400 foot-lamberts.

Since normally bright days will give an average scene luminance of about 900 foot-lamberts, the wearing of sunglasses probably will not improve visual performance much if any at all. In fact, dash-panel readability tests in different automobiles using two subjects who compared no sunglasses with fit-over sunglasses of good quality, and who made over two thousand reaction-time measurements each, showed a 12 percent reduction in performance with the sunglasses in place (Allen, October

1964). Measurements were made on bright summer days. Performance would have been poorer on overcast days, according to the fog room studies just reported.

If glare surfaces of chromium or glossy light-colored paint are in the field of view of a driver the sunglasses may be necessary to achieve comfort, but in the seeing task itself, which is never so bright as glossy metal or paints, no improvement in visual performance is to be expected with sunglasses, and on dull days sunglasses will surely be a visual handicap.

While flying, the sky luminances approach and may exceed the 7,000 foot-lamberts used in the fog room experiment, and relief is needed. At such luminances sunglasses bring a measurable though small increase in visual performance for both far and near tasks and will increase comfort. For flying by far the best performance in quickly recognizing the instrument panel numbers was obtained with a gradient density filter that had about 1 percent transmission at the top and 100 percent transmission in the lower 12-mm. zone of the lens. There is some indication that this lens might be useful in driving. However, such an extreme gradation might be distracting to an earth-bound wearer, especially a pedestrian; to him less extreme gradients might be more acceptable.

An important source of visual degradation due to wearing sunglasses as opposed to clear glasses is the face reflection from the back surface of the dark glass. The special glass will continue to reflect about 4 percent at each surface even though transmission may be very low. Hence reducing the lens transmission is like increasing its surface reflectance. At 4 percent transmission the surface reflection from the back surface will equal the light transmitted, and we have the ingredients for a one-way mirror. For sunglass wear an antireflection coating and dark-colored face skin are distinct visual advantages; they will permit haze-free vision. In military situations it may be beneficial to blacken the skin near the eyes to avoid these reflections. Wrap-around lenses or transparent filter side shields will also help by shading the face near the eyes.

Yellow Lenses

An important but little known feature of yellow sunglasses or shooting glasses is that they fluoresce in daylight (ultraviolet) and scatter a yellow haze over the scene. The haze effect of blue scattered in the atmosphere and of ultraviolet fluorescence in the crystalline lens is replaced by a yellow haze from fluorescing of the glass itself. This undoubtedly accounts in part for the failure of yellow glass to provide the theoretically expected better acuity and performance scores. Generally the scores are the same or worse through such glasses. Some plastics of the Armorlite variety contain an ultraviolet absorbing agent which does not fluoresce (Bailey and Hofstetter, 1959) and should give better vision in daylight than the usual yellow shooting or driving glasses currently available. Fluorescent lights may emit up to 20 percent of their energy in ultraviolet; hence a nonfluorescing ultraviolet filter may be desirable for general wear. Fluorescence of spectacle lenses can be detected with the standard Burton ultraviolet lamp used to view fluorescene patterns in contact lens fitting. The ability of a lens to absorb ultraviolet can be judged by the amount of shading it causes when interposed between the ultraviolet source and a lens or mineral that fluoresces. If the light from the Burton lamp, after passing through a lens to be tested, fails to fluoresce a substance like fluoresene, little if any ultraviolet gets through that lens.

Ultraviolet is of concern because it causes fluorescence of the protein substances in the human eye fluoresce energetically. The visible light thus produced is scattered over the retinal surface and reduces the visibility, especially of small, critical, or poorly illuminated objects.

Cosmetic Tint

The use of the first shade of pink as a cosmetic tint is justified when prescribing rimless eye wear or the nylon-thread-rimmed lenses used in England and Europe. It also can be used to reduce the sometimes serious internal multiple reflections, especially in lenses of minus power, without appreciably affecting transmission in the very thin central portion of the lens.

For lenses in frames and for plus lenses in general there seems to be little justification for a cosmetic tint except for low minus powers to help control internal reflections. Most pink tints in glass absorb ultraviolet efficiently, although some fluoresce. If high intensities of ultraviolet exist in the patient's environment, as out of doors, perhaps pink is justified; otherwise not enough absorption of other wavelengths occurs to make it worthwhile by any other criterion. If the glass fluoresces, the protective absorption of ultraviolet will cause a loss in contrast owing to the visible light scattered from the fluorescing glass.

While little justification can be found for cosmetic tints, there is little harm done by prescribing them for general wear or for day or night driving. The losses in light are only about 5 percent more than the 8-percent loss occurring by surface reflections. Hence a first shade of pink tint in an average prescription power will transmit easily 87 percent of the light. If the surfaces are coated the transmission should rise to about 93 percent.

Ott (April, 1965) has recommended on the basis of a group of plant and animal experiments that ultraviolet is desirable and healthful, and that even window glass as well as spectacles should be made of quartz to pass the ultraviolet. Other researchers cite the proven carcinogenic powers of excessive doses of ultraviolet and its proven ability to age the skin. At the same time it is to be noted that its action upon the skin produces vitamin D, which is necessary for proper calcium metabolism and bone formation.

Little appears to be gained by exposing the eye to ultraviolet, since the cornea stops virtually all of the shorter wavelengths and the lens absorbs or fluoresces the remainder up to 400 nanometers wavelength. None of the ultraviolet penetrates to the retina, and any beneficial effects of ultraviolet must come from its action elsewhere on the body. Certainly the known effects on the eye to date are harmful.

Thermanon, a pale greenish-blue tinted glass similar to ordinary window glass, has been popular as a cataract-preventing lens. Thermanon absorbs both infrared and ultraviolet light energy, and its appearance on the average person is what might be called anticosmetic. It is advertised as a heat-absorbing glass. A modern glass industry found no evidence of the so-called glass blower's cataract among its workers for the past thirty years. It was noted that the employees exposed to the red-hot glass often wore no protective eye wear while the executives and visitors did. Apparently glass blower's cataract must be from some other hazard, perhaps furnace fumes or poisoning from chemicals. Thus the suggested ability of Thermanon to affect the course of a developing cataract is highly speculative.

There are no extensive sources of infrared that the ordinary person could be exposed to that might call for a heat-absorbing glass such as Thermanon. On the other hand, Thermanon absorbs visible red light just as a tinted automobile windshield does and reduces the sensitivity of the wearer to red signals. Combined with a tinted windshield, a Thermanon prescription, especially in plus, would make even the normal driver protanopic. Thus Thermanon or other blue or green glasses should not be prescribed for a driver, pilot, or industrial worker who might depend upon the ability to recognize red quickly for his safety or the safety of others.

WINDSHIELD TINT

Windshield tint conceivably could be a prescription item after the fashion of the fabled Texan who had his spectacle prescription ground into his Cadillac windshield. Windshield tint seems to be considered by the automobile dealers to be essential for all owners of expensive cars and cars with air conditioners; dealer stocks in Bloomington, Indiana, in 1969 were over 95 percent tinted for Oldsmobiles, Pontiacs, Buicks, and Cadillacs. Other manufacturers also used a high percentage of tinted windshields, but not as high as General Motors.

The efficiency of the tint for absorbing the invisible heat rays can never exceed 50 percent, because visible solar energy supplies 50 percent of the heating effect. Once absorbed by the glass the energy elevates the temperature of the glass, which in turn heats the air on both sides of the glass. Hence at best only about 25 percent of the energy hitting the glass can actually be kept out of the car. Since the window area contributes less than 30 percent of the solar heat pickup of the car, and since at best only 25 percent of that, or 7.5 percent, is diverted by the tint in the glass, tint seems an impractical way to control radiation heat uptake, especially since it interferes with vision. A better approach would be to use roof, door, and floor insulation and light-colored exterior paints. A white roof paint plus roof insulation would eliminate at least 44 percent of the solar radiation heat uptake.

Auto manufacturers insist that tint serves to cut discomfort from sitting in the hot sun and that probably this is more important to driver safety than the "small losses" in visibility suffered at night because of the tint. This argument sounded most reasonable until one checked the then existing practice of selling tint only in the windshield. Up until 1969 side windows were never tinted unless air conditioning was ordered, and both a tinted windshield or a tinted windshield plus tinted side windows were and are extra cost items.* If comfort contributes to safety, why is the window next to the driver rarely tinted and why is tinting an extra cost item? The evidence seen in the dealer's inventory stock, in the salesmen's arguments, and in the facts about the low efficiency of tint indicates that tint is more a sales gimmick than a safety or comfort feature; it is not necessary for effective operation of today's adequate air conditioners with local air control, nor is it effective in keeping passengers comfortable in the direct rays of the sun.

Tint might conceivably be prescribed to reduce "glare" in the daytime. However, there is not enough tint to make any comfort difference when 2,000 to 5,000 foot-lamberts of scene brightness needs to be reduced to about 500 foot-lamberts for comfort and maximum seeing efficiency. On the other hand, since the windshield is biased to absorb infrared, it also selectively absorbs the red light from signals and brake lights. This situation is depicted in Figure 8-6. On a bright day where background luminances are high the feeble red signals which are barely adequate at night are further selectively reduced by the tinted windshield. If the patient is also protanopic or protanomalous in his color vision (2 percent of male drivers are) adding windshield tint would be adding to the hazard.

A plate of glass loses light in proportion to its angle to the beam of light (see Figure 8-5). At a 60-degree tilt angle, which is approximately the windshield angle used in American passenger cars, the 70 percent minimum transmission standard for tinted windshields recommended by the Society of Automotive Engineers becomes less than 65 percent. Since a clear windshield at these angles will transmit about 78 percent of the visible light, manufacturers barely pass the SAE code when they use the best clear glass they now make and tilt it to a 60-degree angle. (As far as solar heat and sky light are concerned, these come in nearly normal to

---

* Heat-absorbing glass is in effect clear glass contaminated with iron oxide. In spectacle lenses, at least, untinted glass is more expensive to manufacture.

the surface of the glass, as shown in Figure 8-1.) In this position, heat-absorbing glass will have the least effect in blocking out the harmful or uncomfortable radiation.

One would correctly conclude that the best windshield tint is no tint and the better windshield position is more nearly vertical. One can at least prescribe that the windshield shall not be tinted and shall be kept clean inside and out. If it were possible to order a band of infrared and light-absorbing material in the upper part of the windshield, no lower than 10 degrees above the line of sight of the 90th-percentile driver, this would be desirable. As of the writing of this book there is a hint of possible future government regulation to prevent tint in the lower part of the windshield. At this moment a tinted upper area is automatically accompanied by undesirable uniform tinting over the remainder of the windshield. Hence one cannot prescribe a tinted top band, except by application of spray-on glass tints or plastic panels to the top of the window. The spray-on tints are inconvenient and difficult to use and cannot be recommended for an amateur.

CONTACT LENSES

Contact lenses offer both a benefit and a potential handicap to the driver. Usually visual acuity is not as good with spherical contact lenses as is found with the best spectacle corrections, because of residual astigmatism. Nevertheless, many contact lens patients report they see better than with spectacles, apparently because an unrestricted field of view is offered (and perhaps contact lenses stay cleaner longer, particularly for those who do not regularly wash their spectacles). Cylindrical contact lenses with a spherical back surface and a prism ballast appear to be easy to fit, are comfortable, and provide acuities as good as when spectacles are used.

The spectacle frame is a limiting factor in vision and its removal is a welcome improvement in awareness of everything in the visual field. However, its removal may result in photophobic reactions because the spectacle frame is also a good sun shade. Space distortions from spectacles practically vanish when contact lenses are substituted and the cosmetic improvement for many patients is a benefit worthy of the increased care and patience that the use of contact lenses requires.

NIGHTTIME DRIVING

OPTIMUM PRESCRIPTION LENSES

At night we may have need for a different distance prescription than for the daytime. Night myopia occurs at low levels of illumination at or below that provided by a full moon. There are three components to this phenomenon. First, when the pupil dilates peripheral zones of the cornea and lens are brought into use. Typically these peripheral zones are spherically aberrated positively. Second, at such low levels of illumination the output of the retina seems to be inadequate to hold accommodation accurately on a distant target and accommodation tends to increase. Third, due to the low level of illumination the cones in the retina are dominated by the rods. Since the maximum sensitivity of the rods is about 505 nanometers and that of the cones about 555 nanometers, a shift in the maximum sensitivity toward the blue end of the spectrum occurs, the so-called Purkinje shift. Because the refractive index of the eye increases with shorter wavelengths, the refractive power of the eye increases about 0.50 diopter. These three factors together total about 1.50 diopters increase in refractive power of the eye; that is, about 1.50 diopters of myopia is induced.

A concomitant of night myopia is night presbyopia, which is manifest as a lower and lower measurable amplitude of accommodation as the illumination drops to full night myopia levels.

For patients with low amplitudes of accommodation, say 2.00 diopters or less, only the spherical aberration and chromatic aberration components contribute much to night myopia. For night driving the level of pavement illumination usually exceeds the mesopic vision levels (Richards, August 1967); hence rods never dominate cones. For many patients the pupil size when on the highway at night does not bring in the peripheral zones enough to have a significant effect on refraction. Hence classical night myopia is not present in most driving situations. However, as indicated under the Sensitometric Method of refraction, the eyes of younger people accept less plus than normally prescribed for optimum distance seeing. Thus, one cannot decide for a given patient whether he needs more minus lens power until after he has been tested under actual or simulated night driving conditions.

Because lighting levels fluctuate, one has to have vision commensurate with the dominant type of environment encountered. Unless otherwise indicated the best daytime driving prescription (not sunglasses) is most likely best at night, especially for older persons. The same considerations for youth, uncorrected hyperopia, A.C.A. ratio, etc., as detailed at the beginning of this chapter, apply for nighttime driving as well and may indicate a need for somewhat less plus at night.

LENS REFLECTIONS

Certain powers of spectacle lenses (about +0.50 diopter to −2.00 diopters) are subject to the production of spurious images that are seen clearly by the driver. These images, formed by reflections between the front and back surfaces of the lens, are characteristic of all lenses but are only clearly focused on the retina in lenses near zero power, especially on the minus side. For these few it is virtually mandatory that the lenses be antireflection coated. A cosmetic tint is of some help, but the antireflection coating is the procedure of choice. These reflections should be of no concern in sunglasses. Sometimes the corneal reflex itself is mirrored by a lens surface so as to be clearly focused on the retina. This can be corrected easily by changing the lens distance from the eye, changing the height of the lens, or tilting it.

YELLOW LENSES

"Night driving" lenses have been shown to provide no benefit in seeing ability at night (Richards 1964). They are even hazardous, because they give the driver a feeling of seeing better which no one has yet been able to explain (Septon, 1968). Studies have shown that they actually impair visual performance and retard glare recovery. Many promoters have made unfounded claims for the ability of amber to improve night vision. They often employ mass solicitation, usually by mail. The Federal Trade Commission has correctly ruled that such practices are illegal since the lenses do not perform as claimed.

CONTACT LENSES

Contact lenses have some problems for nighttime wear of importance to drivers. The most popular are the corneal contact lenses which are about 8 mm. in diameter and float on a film of tears near the center of the cornea. The optical zone is usually about 6 mm. in diameter. Often the edge and peripheral transition zone near the edge of these lenses can cause a ring of light or a circular shadow to be seen around objects. At night the pupil may enlarge to 7 mm., which is larger than the optical zone of the contact lens, and lights will appear to have a flare or blur around them owing to the edge of the contact lens.

To be sure that the lenses are large enough for night as well as day wear, a diurnal study of the pupil size should be run. This can be done with a subjective pupil gauge (see Figure 6-11) with which the patient can measure his own pupil at several times during the twenty-four-hour period and report the results. The contact lens optical zone should be at least the same size as the largest pupil encountered. Hence, if the patient reports a 7-mm. pupil on the highway at night, the optical zone diameter should be at least 7 mm. This will ensure that the edge blur is well outside the central field of view under most driving conditions.

Contact lenses must be kept free of oily deposits, since failure to wet the surface of the plastic will degrade the retinal image and lower visual performance, especially at night-driving levels of luminance. If a suitably large lens that remains clean and wetted throughout the wearing period cannot be found, the patient should not wear contact lenses for night driving. Of course, there may be serious spectacle problems at night as well, in which case it may be prudent to recommend no driving at night.

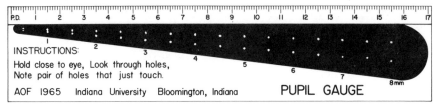

Figure 6-11. Pupil measuring device. Pinholes spaced at one half millimeter intervals permit the selection of the pair that are seen to just touch when held close before the eye. Since the image on the retina of a point object placed very close before the eye is blurred, the limit of the blur-circle size is the size of the pupil of the eye. When their two blur-circle images are tangent to one another, point objects in the anterior focal plane of the eye must of necessity be spaced a distance apart equal to the diameter of the entrance pupil. (The principles involved in this P.D. gauge are not original with the author.)

Bifocal contact lenses should be evaluated for the degree of interference occurring with the larger pupil usually found with night driving. A simple test consisting of a bare flashlight bulb without a reflector exposed to the patient at twenty feet in a dark room will give a good indication. Allow three minutes for the pupil to achieve approximately its full size. If the segment will cause glare, haze, or halo problems, then an excessive amount of streaking, halo or hazing will appear around the point of light. The type of light scatter displayed will vary with the design and placement of the segment and with the pupil size. It is wise to have the subject move his eyes, as in driving, to determine the effect of lens lag upon the scattered light.

COSMETIC TINT

For nighttime use a cosmetic tint (such as CxA or Soft Lite #1) does not seem to present a significant hazard. The 5 percent loss due to the tint provides some benefit by reducing the ghost images produced by reflections between the lens surfaces. Antireflection coating on a cosmetic tint would provide an overall transmission somewhat greater than that of uncoated clear glass. Thermanon, on the other hand, cannot be recommended because of its reduced transmission, especially of red light, and because its absorption adds to the absorption in tinted windshields.

WINDSHIELD TINT

If you prescribe a tinted windshield for night driving you are in effect telling your patient to turn off at least one of his headlights with respect to the light returned to his eyes from the roadway. Of course, it also will reduce headlight glare by an equal amount, which can deceive you into thinking you have improved seeing. But consider what happens if we carry this to the ultimate limit with darker and darker windshield tints. The last thing you will be able to see as the tint is increased will be the glare sources themselves. Let's go the other way instead and remove all tint and start adding more light to the environment (which your own headlights do). The ultimate would be full daytime brightnesses, whereupon "glaring" headlights no longer are very glaring even when one looks directly at them. Thus the tinted windshield offers only increased hazard at night.

Perhaps the greatest hazard posed by the tinted windshield is to pedestrians. Every driver with tinted windows knows that when he's looking for a house number at night, he rolls down his window to see better. Pedestrians are noted for wearing dark clothing and unexpectedly appearing as if out of nowhere. Unfortunately, windshields cannot be rolled down to permit greater visibility as one can do when looking for house numbers. The typical driver statement in nighttime pedestrian accidents is "I didn't see him" or "I didn't see him until he was right in front of my car and I couldn't stop." Most victims at night are adults; in the daytime they include children, too. The typical daytime comment is "He darted into the street." Since more than 10,000 pedestrians are killed each year and most of these deaths occur at night, one wonders about the argument that the daytime benefits of tinted windshields outweigh their increased hazard at night.

A tinted windshield cannot even be sold safely as a prescription item for a given person because it is likely that the car will be driven by others. If a tinted windshield is installed, it should be labeled as hazardous for driving at night and for color-defective drivers.

WINDSHIELD REFLECTIONS

One of the most annoying windshield defects shows up at night as doubled lights due to internal reflections in the glass. These are present in the daytime, too, and serve to reduce contrast and to permit greater spread of the light from glare sources. The doubling effect can be seen in the daytime by looking at the glare reflected from chromium. At night approaching automobiles typically will have an accompanying line of ghost headlights nearby. Red tail lights will have an ethereal red ghost floating near them. Multiple internal reflections of the windshield will not produce visible ghost images if the surfaces are parallel for flat glass and properly wedged for bent glass. A driver patient reporting double vision might have a monocular refractive, or a binocular fusional, problem, a set of in-focus reflections from his glasses, a poor-quality windshield, or even images produced by a highly polished hood.

WINDSHIELD AGE

A review of the literature reveals no evidence that windshield aging studies have been carried out on motor vehicles on the highway. When the plastic layer in the middle of the windshield sandwich was chosen it was investigated for aging, but the aging of the glass itself seems not to have been considered. That glass deteriorates is reported by drivers in desert regions where sandstorms occur and where wipers act on a layer of abrasive dust during window washer operation. Little attention has been paid to the deterioration caused by the energetic station attendant using various bug cleaning methods or just grinding the road dust into the glass with a paper towel as is done in wintertime in below freezing weather.

Windshield deterioration first came to the author's attention when he found that he could not clean a three-year-old windshield. After trying several solvents he inspected the glass itself by focusing on it as a set of headlights approached at night. A beautiful series of circular rings appeared centered about the lights and extended across virtually the entire windshield. These scratches were not concentric with the wiper arm axle but with the light itself. This indicated a random series of microscopic scratches in the glass, probably caused by the circular movements used in hand-cleaning the glass. A most dramatic improvement in the ability to see against the oncoming headlights occurred by leaning out the side window and looking around the windshield. Instantly there was no glare. The roadway ahead was seen easily and the approaching headlights caused no difficulties or discomfort.

A new windshield did not cause this glare problem. By looking at windshields on a bright day one can see that a new windshield produces a clean-margined image of the reflection of the sun while an old windshield has a concentric ring pattern, causing the sun's image to expand onto the adjacent glass. Of course, a dirty windshield causes a haze to extend across the windshield, but without the bright hairline scratches concentrically oriented.

The optometrist whose patient complains of glare or annoyance in driving, even after he has received a new pair of glasses, should arrange to inspect the windshield and headlights of the patient's car (see Figure 6-12). If any vehicular problems exist, it should be easy to demonstrate to the owner the wisdom of a new windshield, better headlight aim, and greater cleanliness of head lamps, tail lamps and windows.

HEADLIGHT AIM

The percentage of cars with less than the full complement of headlights, with headlights improperly aimed, with headlights covered by a generous layer of dirt, or with sleepy eye shields over the top half of the lamps (see Figure 8-14), is very great. It is to be hoped that mandatory vehicle inspection being adopted by all states will make it clear to the driving public that headlights are an important part of safe nighttime driving. The usual argument against driving with one headlight out is that other drivers cannot determine whether they are approaching a car or a motorcycle. Actually, an equally realistic problem is the loss in illumination that accompanies the loss of a headlight.

Glare is a problem in contrast. If you try to look into the window of a house in the daytime you find it impossible because the amount of light reflected from the outside wall is greater than that from inside the house. (Yet, that same amount of inside light is quite adequate for vision as soon as you enter, leaving the high luminance levels outside.) In effect the outside wall is so glaring that you can't see objects as dimly lighted as those normally found in a house in the daytime.

At night there is little light from the outside of the house and it is easy to see in, even though there is only a fraction of the luminance available in the house. Similarly, at night, approaching automobile headlights

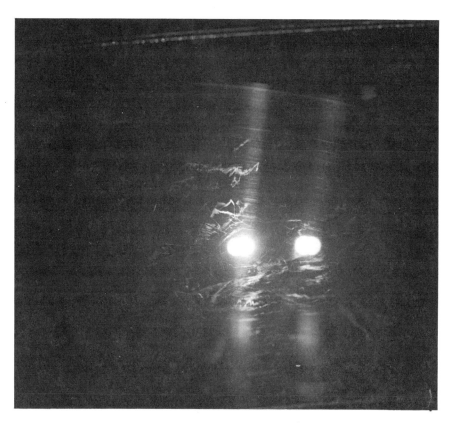

Figure 6-12. Windshield deterioration. A windshield removed and photographed after 102,349 miles of driving in the Toledo, Ohio, region. The radial pattern is from the wipers while the zigzag patterns are from scraping the surface with a hard substance such as metal. Obviously the effect of the glare of oncoming headlights is greatly extended by such windshield damage.

would reduce vision like the bright outside wall of the house. By adding some light to the night scene from your own automobile headlights, the contrast of the approaching lights is reduced and vision is improved. Headlights must be aimed to avoid glare to others, and must also provide as much illumination on the roadway, and as far forward, as possible. Properly aimed headlights that are dirty become glaring to others and, because of a reduced ability to light the roadway due to the dirt, make oncoming headlights by contrast seem more glaring still.

The optometrist should recommend a careful headlight alignment and the maintenance of clean headlight lenses free of amber filters, half shields, or other gimmickry that reduces the light output or spoils the designed output distribution. Next to a good prescription to provide clear, comfortable vision, good headlight aim and clean lights and windows are the most important solutions to glare at night. Under certain conditions it may prove desirable to recommend halogen driving lights, or white lens fog lamps, or the Chrysler Super-Lite for use in freeway driving and in light traffic for two-lane night driving. Only the Super-Lite can be safely used on two-lane roads with approaching traffic because of its extremely circumscribed pattern and sharp cutoff, yet it about doubles the seeing range against oncoming headlights. The recommendation that more light be used only when there is no danger of overpowering the vision of other drivers is an excellent solution to some of the seeing problems at night. If all automobiles had more headlight power, the highways would be safer at night.

Chapter 7: Drivers with Special Visual Problems

SQUINT

VARIOUS ESTIMATES place the incidence of squint in the population at from 2 to 7 percent. Many authorities consider a squinter to be the equivalent of a one-eyed person, which is certainly not the case. The squinting eye is relied upon for peripheral vision and in some cases it alternates, taking turns with the other eye for "normal" seeing.

The abnormal eye position of a squinter is almost always a result of perceptual adaptation to help him live with double vision. Under anaesthesia half of all squinters are straight (Reinecke and Miller, 1966). Under abnormal stress situations the squint angle has been observed to change radically, which would displace the retinal image from its usual squint angle position on the retina of the deviating eye. This is an excellent way to cause a squinter to see double. At low levels of illumination under stresses such as fatigue, alcohol, carbon monoxide, and ill health, the adaptations that protect the squinter from double vision and confusion may be lost. Hence no squinter should be assumed to be a completely safe driver until it is demonstrated that he cannot be induced to see double under any condition.

The majority of unoperated squinters are well adapted to their condition and do not often become visually confused, but this does not preclude the possibility that they might behave like a binocular person with a misaligned eye under certain conditions. The post-surgical squinter has a more serious problem which may affect his ability to drive safely. He is probably still a squinter but one whose perceptual adaptation has been destroyed by a surgical change in squint angle. Surgical success in accomplishing binocular vision, even with the aid of medical orthoptics as currently practiced, is less than one out of every seven patients. Most squint treatment by surgery is intended to achieve at least a cosmetic cure, which is achieved in about 80 percent of the patients. Because the great bulk of all squinters do not have a muscle problem (Adler, 1965, p. 524),

78

the patient's eyes usually do not stay where the muscle surgery places them. A series of operations is thus scheduled, each on a different muscle (Reinicke et al, 1964) until the eyes remain within ±15Δ of straight. This is a cosmetic cure. New scar tissue and adhesions are formed with each surgical intervention, motility is impaired, and the patient (usually a child) is left with diplopia, limited ocular motility, and a squint angle that varies with the direction of gaze, a most distressing situation. Should we give him a driver's license when he is old enough?

The following quotation by Ruedeman (1953), a well known American ophthalmologist, will give us an indication of what we can expect of some our citizens who have been cured of squint by surgery.

> Over a period of years, keeping very accurate studies of the end results of ocular muscle surgery, I have been embarrassed and chagrined many times by the tendency of the foveas to revert to their previous positions. The central vision in the operated eye is not maintained and, although the youngster is somewhat improved, many are unable to carry on in school at an intelligence level equal to their age and normal social group.
>
> There has been, and is, something drastically missing in our handling of the normal so-called muscle problem. Over a period of years, the records of these cases have been reported visually in a photographic way without records as to their fusional end results, not taken at periods long enough after the surgery has been instituted, to warrant listing them as cures.
>
> From this study of my own statistics, for the sake of the record, I might say that I have cosmetically straightened 80% of my cases, at least giving them a good anatomic correction. This is truly a cosmetic result and has little to do with the physio-psychological intellectual level of the individual upon whom this operation has been performed. By chance, and with some orthoptic treatment, about 10% of this group has been held in 2nd grade fusion and less than 10% in 3rd grade fusion.
>
> It was my contention as long as 20 years ago that, unless we carried these patients completely to 3rd grade fusion and unless they could hold this fusion over long enough periods of time with good fusional amplitude, we were developing our own group of neurotics, our own group of people who had nervous breakdowns, and people with inferior intellectual abilities.
>
> The key to successful re-education is to build an individual's use of the foveas, which means an early diagnosis and reeducation to precede and follow the muscle surgery, if that is necessary, which in reality is only a means of interrupting the faulty eye-brain pattern.

An untreated squinter of driving age usually is visually well adapted and, except to the extent that society has ridiculed and made fun of him, he will be competent in most situations. Squinters of long duration are usually so well adapted to their condition that they have great difficulty accepting normal binocular vision even when the surgeon provides him with reasonably straight eyes.

Unfortunately the more hazardous surgically treated group will not be obvious to the motor vehicle driver license examiner, while the probably safe untreated squinter will usually be easy to detect. The examiner, upon noting a deviating eye or learning of eye surgery for a deviation of the eyes, should restrict driving to daytime low-stress situations, unless the applicant has been certified by an optometrist or ophthalmologist as being safe to drive.

Squinters cured by nonsurgical means can be considered normal. In work at the Optometric Center of New York, William Ludlam (1961) found that the cure rate was 73 percent for squinters who had not had surgery. The criteria of cure (Flom, 1958) were so rigid that these former squinters could not be identified upon routine optometric examination if the case history were omitted!

SUPPRESSION

Suppression of vision in one eye when both eyes are open often accompanies squint and should be subject to the same precautions about driving. If suppression accompanies a nondeviating ocular condition, such as aniseikonia with peripheral fusion, it probably is not a hazard of any significance, although the subject will not have stereopsis. He probably could not operate safely in close situations such as required of school bus drivers, truckers, crane operators, fork lift operators, or operators of road building equipment. However, ordinary high-speed highway driving probably relies very little on stereopsis except when traffic densities are high on multiple-lane highways.

AMBLYOPIA

Amblyopia is a condition of reduced acuity in one eye and it may or may not be associated with a squint. Like suppression, it is an adaptation and poses no special problem so long as a squint does not exist and peripheral fusion is present. The remarks above on the lack of stereopsis associated with suppression pertain also to amblyopia.

ANISOCORIA

A difference in pupil size between the two eyes of a clinically significant amount occurs in about 17 percent of the population. Pathology should always be suspected in anisocoria. The anisocoria may disappear as the patient recovers from the pathology. If the anisocoria is permanent, it may be desirable to prescribe a compensating spectacle filter before one eye, to dilate the normal eye, or to prescribe a filter contact lens over the large pupil eye.

A difference in pupil size will cause a difference in retinal illumination which will cause a stereoscopic judgment error for moving targets. This stereoscopic effect, the Pulfrich stereo phenomenon (Lit, 1966), can be produced also by glare entering only one eye, by an uncorrected difference in refraction, or by a difference in retinal image size. Other sources of differences leading to Pulfrich stereo effects are uniocular beginning cataract, a cloudy vitreous, vitreous or aqueous floaters, and retinal abnormalities.

The Pulfrich stereo phenomenon causes illusions affecting the apparent location, speed of movement, and size of objects seen while driving and could lead to collision situations. Figure 7-1 shows that the perceptual delay caused by reduced retinal illumination in the left eye will cause an automobile moving to the right across the highway to be seen farther away. Illusions also occur as one moves along the roadway in an automobile. If one looks straight ahead, objects on the right move farther to the right as they come closer, while objects on the left move to the left. According to Figure 7-1, an object moving to the right is seen farther away if the left eye has a reduced retinal illumination. Of course, objects moving to the left would appear closer.

While driving, objects on either side of the roadway appear to move farther to the side as we move past them. The images of the objects move across the retina at their proper velocities and proper sizes, but because they appear to be at abnormal distances, due to image brightness differences, the observer with anisocoria as illustrated reports the following: Objects on the right appear to be larger than normal and to move at a slower rate; those on the left appear to be smaller and to zip by at an alarming rate. When rounding a curve, the speed and distance distortions are rather startling and lead to a feeling of insecurity. In fact, all five drivers who wore a 20 percent transmission gray filter over one eye on a winding rural Indiana road for thirty minutes became carsick.

To see the effect of the Pulfrich phenomenon upon normal driving, take a tour slowly through the local neighborhood and at normal speeds on the highway. Wear a pair of dark sunglasses (about 20 percent transmission) with one lens removed. In the first five minutes or so there probably will be little noticeable effect of the brightness imbalance between the eyes. Slowly the awareness of the difference in speed between the right and left sides of the street will develop, followed closely by marked size differences and finally by road slant. If worn enough a feeling of insecurity and perhaps even nausea may develop.

A most fascinating illusion occurs when wearing a unilateral filter while walking or riding very slowly. For example, sit in your automobile in your driveway and look out your side window at the ground. Drive the car forward *very slowly* for a few feet, stop gently, and reverse direction for a few feet. Depending on the eye that is covered with the filter,

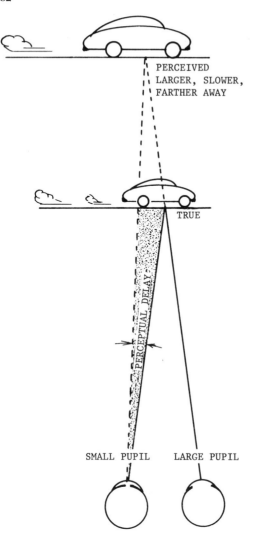

Figure 7-1. Schematic representation of the effect of reducing
the illumination in the left eye.
The small pupil in the left eye
reduces the retinal illumination
and causes a delayed perception
from the left eye.

the ground will appear close or far away, and vegetation along the driveway will shrink or enlarge to surprising proportions. A hedge becomes a
forest of trees or is tiny as if viewed from the top of the house!

It seems unlikely that adaptation can occur to these aberrations of
space. Since the illusions depend upon both the velocity and direction of
motion across the retina, the adaptation, if it could occur, would require
a long time and probably would never be complete. Both the spatial distortion effects and the nausea observed during our studies indicate that
differential retinal image brightness should be of concern in tending the

visual needs of the motoring public. One method of handling involves the prescription of a filter over the eye with the brighter image. This filter is chosen by viewing at five meters a swinging pendulum or a rotating disc as described in Chapter 5. Any falsely perceived circular pendulum motion or tilt of the rotating disc can be neutralized by filters placed before the eye with the greater transmission.

To equate the retinal luminances, sunglass filters of about 50 percent transmission used singly or in combination will provide fine enough increments to permit useful measurements. One must keep in mind that a daytime correction may become a nighttime error, because the pupils may become equal (or unequal) upon dilation in the dark. Thus, it may be necessary to wear a different balancing filter, one for day and one for night use. Because of the cosmetic problem created by a uniocular filter, the use of Neo-synephrine to dilate the smaller pupil or eserine to constrict the larger pupil might be a method of choice. Since the drug actions cannot be precisely controlled and since there may be contraindications to the use of drugs over prolonged periods of time, only large pupil size differences may be suited for this approach.

The use of an 0.50- to 0.75-diopter fogging lens over the weaker eye may be sufficient to destroy stereopsis and eliminate the space-distorting effects of the differences in pupil size. Since this has not been clinically reported as a successful method and since there are important contraindications, it should be approached with caution.

Contact lenses of differing transmission appear to be acceptable both cosmetically and functionally to correct a transmission difference between the eyes, whatever may be the cause of that difference. Of course, the Pulfrich stereo phenomenon requires good binocular vision with stereopsis, and, if stereopsis is not present, it is not necessary to consider a correction for brightness differences between the eyes.

ANISEIKONIA

Differences in retinal image size up to 5 percent appear to be clinically unimportant for most people. For differences of 5 percent and over, patients may suffer significant space distortions, double vision, tropias, headaches, nausea, and disorientation. Aniseikonia causes space distortions only for people who have good binocular vision with stereopsis, and large amounts (over approximately 15 percent) preclude binocular vision, leading to amblyopia, suppression, or squint.

During daytime hours, multiple clues to space help maintain proper orientation for uncorrected aniseikonic patients. However, when only points of light and limited roadway illumination are present, as at night, the effects of aniseikonia may become serious. Aniseikonia can cause stereo displacements for objects moving across the retina just as does a filter placed before one eye. It also causes various major effects such as ground tilt to the left or right or an uphill or downhill tilt, depending on the type of aniseikonia. The patient may compensate adequately when he is fully rested, but he will have increasing difficulty under conditions of low illumination, fatigue, alcohol, carbon monoxide, or other physiological stressors.

It appears that the small aniseikonic differences between old and new spectacles are the source of new-spectacle annoyance which may require up to two weeks for patient adaptation. That patients can adapt is of interest, for it implies a functional shifting of corresponding points on the two retinas, a phenomenon supported by other types of data. Furthermore, the small percentage of aniseikonic patients found in the average practice indicates a high degree of neurological adaptability of the human being to optical differences, both natural ones and those induced by spectacles. This suggests that aniseikonic patients and patients receiving new eye wear might respond more quickly if one instituted binocular stereoscopic, ocular motility and Bartley enhancement flash frequency types of training to restructure more quickly the neurological interconnections responsible for retinal correspondence.

One serious consequence of prescribing large aniseikonic corrections is an increase in spectacle distortion. Size-difference corrections are obtained by steepening or flattening the base curves on one lens, by increasing the thickness of one lens, and by changing the distance of the placement of one of the lenses in front of the eyes relative to the other lens. As a result the optimum prescription correction from edge to center is lost, and increasing distortions are noticed. Distortions themselves are, in effect, nonlinear aniseikonic errors which, like the Pulfrich phenomenon, are not easy to adapt to. Whenever a choice exists, base curves should be steepened rather than flattened to reduce distortions. Eye wear that provides secure placement of the lenses should be chosen to prevent abnormal pantoscopic angles or downward displacement due to mishandling by the patient. Alignment of spectacles to the face should be done by aligning the line of sight and the lens surface reflections as indicated in Figures 6-1 through 6-10.

CYCLOPHORIA

The measurement of cyclophoria is often neglected because most practitioners feel that nothing can be done about it. Very few clinic cases are reported in the literature except in association with squint, and its importance in drivers' vision is little understood. Cyclophoria tends to cause a vertical doubling on either side of the fovea and stereopsis errors for objects above and below the fovea. The average person has about 1 degree of excyclophoria at distance. If only 2 minutes of excyclo-disparity exists during binocular vision, a street light one hundred meters away and six meters above the roadway will appear to be six meters nearer than the point on the roadway immediately beneath the light. If, under low levels of illumination, the excyclo-disparity increases, the error in localizing the street light will increase alarmingly.

Though there are no practical prescribable lenses capable of rotating the image around the line of sight, one can confidently undertake ocular motility training to reduce or eliminate the cyclophoria. Training of ocular motility and of lateral fusional amplitudes in general will indirectly strengthen vertical and cycloduction ability. Cyclofusional training per se can be given in a synoptophore type of instrument, a stereoscope, or another form of haploscope where the targets can be manipulated separately. Cycloductions can be expected to improve if rotation training is given throughout the ranges of normal ocular motility. A simple direct trainer is a vertical piece of string viewed against a uniform background, or a vertical line on a twelve-inch disc. When the subject holds either target at about thirteen inches from his eyes with the line vertical and views it binocularly, incyclofusion is stimulated when the line is tilted top toward the patient, and excyclofusion is stimulated when the top is tilted away. Cyclofusional movements are like vertical fusional movements in that they occur very slowly. Thus, cyclofusional doubling will occur sooner if the stimulus is increased rapidly.

COLOR BLINDNESS

Normal color vision is called *trichromatism* because three primary colors can be mixed to match every possible perceived color. Color "blindness" commonly includes the anomalous trichromats as well as the dichromats and monochromats. An excellent analysis of color vision types and characteristics is given in the following table (Judd, 1943):

TABLE 7-1

CLASSIFICATION AND CHARACTERISTICS OF THE VARIOUS COLOR VISION SYSTEMS

Type, number of components	Discriminations possible	Maximum luminosity, nm	Neutral points, nm	Nontheoretical v. Kries	Designations		
					Young-Helmholtz	*Hering*	*G. E. Muller*
Trichromatism	Light-dark Yellow-blue Red-green	555	None	Normal system	Normal system	Normal system	Normal system
	Light-dark Yellow-blue Red-green (weak)	540	None	Protanomaly[1]	Abnormal red function	—	Alteration[4] system
	Light-dark Yellow-blue Red-green (weak)	560	None	Deuteranomaly[1]	Abnormal green function	Red-green weakness	Alteration[4] system
	Light-dark Red-green Yellow-blue (weak)	560	None	Tritanomaly[2]	Abnormal violet function	Yellow-blue weakness	Alteration[4] system
Dichromatism	Light-dark Yellow-blue	540	493	Protanopia[6]	Red blindness	—	Outer red-green blindness
	Light-dark Yellow-blue	560	497	Deuteranopia[6]	Green blindness	Red-green blindness	Inner red-green blindness

Light-dark Red-green	560	572	Tritanopia	Violet blindness	—	Outer yellow-blue blindness
Light-dark Red-green	560	470 580	Tetartanopia [3]	—	Yellow-blue blindness	Inner yellow-blue blindness
Monochromatism Light-dark	510	All	Congenital total color-blindness [7]	—	—	Cone blindness [5]
Light-dark	560	All	Acquired total color-blindness	—	Total color blindness	Inner total color blindness, Type I
Light-dark	540	All	—	—	—	Inner total color blindness, Type II

[1] Konig proposed the designation *anomalous trichromatism* for the classes later designated separately by Nagel in an extension of the v. Kries terminology.

[2] This extension of the v. Kries terminology was proposed by Engelking.

[3] This extension of the v. Kries terminology was proposed by Muller.

[4] The term *alteration system* was proposed originally by v. Kries; Muller also uses Nagel's terminology.

[5] The term *cone blindness* is based upon the duplicity theory of v. Kries and Parinaud, now widely accepted.

[6] Protanopic observers are sometimes called *scoterythrous;* and deuteranopic, *photerythrous.*

[7] Total color blindness is often called *achromatopsia* or *achromatopia.*

The incidence of the various types of color vision defects for male and female members of the population is given in the following table (Judd, 1943).

TABLE 7-2
FREQUENCY OF OCCURRENCE
OF INHERITED VISUAL SYSTEMS

Number of Components	Designation Nontheoretical	Percentage of the Population Male	Female
Anomalous trichromatism	Protanomaly	1.0	0.02
	Deuteranomaly	4.9	0.38
	Tritanomaly	0.0001	0.0000
		5.9	0.40
Dichromatism	Protanopia	1.0	0.02
	Deuteranopia	1.1	0.01
	Tritanopia	0.0001	0.0000
	Tetartanopia	0.0001	0.0000
		2.1	0.03
Monochromatism	Total color blindness	0.003	0.002
	Abnormal systems	8.0	0.43
	Normal system	92.0	99.57

An important consideration in color vision is the sensitivity of the eye to various wavelengths of light. Protanomaly and protanopia are both clearly different from the normal in this respect, while most other color vision defects have wavelength sensitivities which are more or less normal. See Figure 7-2.

Color vision may be further classified as acquired or inherited. Acquired color vision defects are said to accompany diseases affecting the retina, nerve pathways, or visual cortex. Significant among these are multiple sclerosis, optic neuritis, pernicious anemia, leukemia, vitamin deficiency, diabetes, and retinopathies. Toxic amblyopia has an accompanying color defect. Among the causes of toxic amblyopia are carbon disulfide, lead, certain of the antibiotics, iodoform, thallium (rat poison and depilatory), and, most common of all, tobacco (including snuff) and alcohol.

Inherited color vision defects are widely believed to account for the bulk of color vision problems. Successful research has been concentrated on finding the inherited photopigment defects presumed to be present in the various color anomalies.

"Normal" color vision is only normal under special conditions. For example, parafoveal vision resembles deuteranomaly, intermediate peripheral vision resembles deuteranopia, while extreme periphery resembles monochromatism. In the parafoveal region it is possible to see small lights whose area is insufficient to elicit a color sensation, thus resembling monochromatism. At luminance levels which are below the knee in the dark adaptation curve, the normal eye behaves as if it were totally color-blind. During short or repetitive flashes of light the normal color sensation may not develop, or it develops in a highly abnormal manner dependent upon the color of the flash, the frequency, the light-dark interval, and the surround. A temporary color perception aberration occurs following preadaptation to a given color or exposure of a color in an extensive colored surround.

Some evidence exists that at least some anomalous trichromats are not defective at all but yet are different from "normals." The dichromats and monochromats are currently thought to be defectives in one way or another. Though there is strong evidence that photopigments can be defective or abnormal, there is also increasing evidence of an important neurological aspect to color vision.

A review of current electrophysiological research reports indicates that some color vision anomalies, especially of the anomalous trichro-

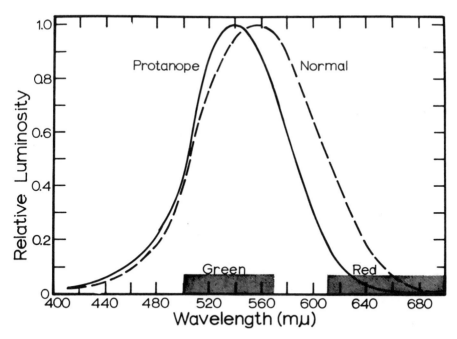

Figure 7-2. Relative sensitivities of protanopic color-blind and normal color vision persons. Those wavelengths that could be called green or red are indicated by the bars along the abscissa.

matic type, might better be named *color amblyopias* and that training techniques appropriate to amblyopia might be successfully applied. During World War II many attempts were made to train color defectives. No systematic studies using anomaloscopes or colorimeters were run on the majority of those trained; hence claims of success were generally unsubstantiated. Efforts at training were simple and were usually without the benefit of knowledge of even what type of anomaly was being treated. I predict that the deuteranomalous group, 2.62 percent of the population, will show the greatest response to training while the protanopic and monochromatic groups will be least responsive, if at all, to training. Ball and Bartley (1967) have already shown that color perception can be changed temporarily from normal to anomalous and vice versa in the laboratory, indicating a strong neurological aspect to the perception of color.

From the above it is apparent that color is not a safe way to impart information to all drivers. Shape coding is absolutely essential. The reliance upon red is unfortunate in view of the difficulties in seeing red by the protanomalous and protanopic observers who, combined, total 2.04 percent of the population. Since females account for the .04 percent and since males do most of the driving, it is obvious that nearly 4 percent of the drivers on our roads at an average time are relatively *very insensitive to red*.

A driver who knows he has a defect and the nature of the hazard it creates will probably be more careful; hence color vision tests and counseling for those who are defective should be routine for all drivers.

GLAUCOMA

Glaucoma is characterized by depression of visual function and progressing field scotomata. When treated with miotics to lower the intraocular pressure, a reduced retinal illumination and a reduction in retinal sensitivity result, owing to direct action of the miotic on the retina. Iris nodules and a predisposition toward cataract has been noted to accompany prolonged use of miotics. Both the visual field defects, the reduction of light transmission, and the reduction of retinal sensitivity contraindicate driving at night. Windshield tint is especially contraindicated for glaucoma patients receiving daily eye drops. Headlights should be clean and properly aimed and have their light output boosted with a relay to improve nighttime vision.

If glaucoma can be controlled with diet or medications other than miotics, there should be little problem driving at night so long as the visual fields remain normal. Uniocular miotic treatment for glaucoma can cause serious space distortions due to the Pulfrich stereo effect and should be avoided whenever alternatives are possible.

ALBINISM

A true albino has no retinal or iris pigment and has a very poor contrast sensitivity, has poor visual acuity, and is color-blind. However, complete albinism is rare. An albino probably could not demonstrate the needed acuity to drive an automobile, but if he did pass the vision test he should drive only with extreme caution. A contact lens that shades the sclera as well as the iris should markedly improve contrast sensitivity and glare resistance and may make some albinos into safe drivers in bright daylight. An albino should be given a performance test under typical driving conditions before being allowed full driving freedom. Visual treatment for albinism should begin within a few days or weeks after birth to avoid the permanent neurological deficit that makes the benefit of the fitting of pinhole contact lenses so marginal in the adult. Treatment consists of supplying a clear retinal image for at least an hour each day in early infancy by means of widely spaced pinholes in an occluder until the infant is old enough to wear contact lenses with dark portions covering the sclera and outer portions of the cornea.

RETINITIS AND UVEITIS

Acute inflammatory processes will be characterized by abnormalities in color perception, critical fusion frequency, visual acuity, and contrast sensitivity. Vitreous floaters and blood cells in the aqueous may reduce vision to finger counting in a day or so. Sometimes a person may not be fully aware of a chronic ocular pathology. Such people should be under the care of a physician and should not drive until given permission to do so. Usually permission to drive in the daytime will be granted first, as the patient recovers.

Chronic internal ocular disease may or may not produce marked abnormalities of perception. Visual field defects or reduced acuity may be enough to prevent the patient from holding a driving license. Individual patients may be able to drive quite well by day, but few will be able to drive safely at night. Certainly these people also should be under the care of a physician. Low vision aids which increase the image size at distance also cause unacceptable field defects. These aids cannot improve visual performance significantly at low illumination levels.

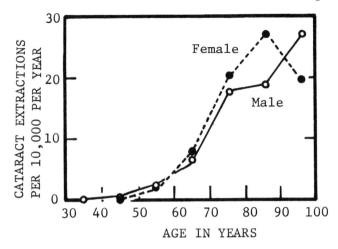

Figure 7-3. Age of first extraction of a cataract per 10,000 at risk per year (Pirie, 1968).

PHOTOPHOBIA

Unusual sensitivity to light, or photophobia, varies from vague discomfort to copious tearing and blepharospasm. Uncorrected refractive errors, aphakia, albinism, and dilated pupils are common causes of photophobia. Sun burning of the cornea or conjunctiva or the presence of an iritis produces a painful photophobia. Central nervous system abnormalities due to disease, angiospasm, minor stroke, or nutritional deficiencies, or similar problems at the retinal level, are often accompanied by photophobia. Cataracts may produce photophobic symptoms in the early stages owing to light scattered within the eye and to fluorescence of the lens in blue light.

Some protection from the discomfort of photophobia is provided by sunglasses, which should transmit about 30 percent and should be neutral gray in color. Losses in the red end of the spectrum occur when green lenses are worn, and some green and blue lenses make the wearer effectively protanopic if he wasn't to begin with. Yellow or amber lenses heighten the photophobic reaction of most people at high luminances.

Photophobia induced by headlights at night *must not* be treated with sunglasses or a tinted windshield. First, the optometrist should suspect a scratched and dirty windshield. Second, the headlights are likely to be misaligned or partially inoperative and dirty. When photophobia appears to be unusually acute, a nutritional, toxic, or pathological condition might be the cause. Referral for a medical check-up and nutritional evaluation is quite proper. Such a step may also result in stopping or reversing an early cataract formation. The Alpascope (Hofstetter, January 1968) may be helpful in assessing the normalcy of a patient's reaction to high-intensity glare sources and for evaluating improvements which may occur with such treatments as may be found necessary by the examining physician.

CATARACT

"Nearly everyone over 55 has peripheral spokes or opacities in the lens, yet even in the age group having the highest rate of cataract extraction (women of over 75 years of age), only 0.3% per year do in fact have a cataract of sufficient severity to need removal " (Pirie, 1968).

TABLE 7-3
CLASSIFICATION OF EXTRACTED HUMAN CATARACTS
(*Pirie, 1968*)

Group	Characteristics of Lens	Percent
I	Uniform pale yellow	45
II	Pale cortex with visible nucleus	42
III	Pale cortex with hazel brown nucleus	11
IV	Pale cortex with deep brown nucleus	2

From Table 7-3 we may infer that 45 percent of all beginning cataracts are apt to be of the diffuse type without a central nucleus and that presumably such a cataract would grow mostly from the periphery in. Thus roughly one half of the cataracts will give good daytime vision (peripheral cataract) and the other half good nighttime vision (central cataract) in the early stages. Figure 7-3 shows the incidence of first cataract surgery per 10,000 population per year in England. Presumably cataract surgery would be delayed until acuities below 20/40 had developed and were handicapping the patient in driving, reading, and other activities.

Figure 7-4 shows the number of drivers by age and sex in the United States in 1966. About 20 million drivers were fifty-five and older. By assuming that the British experience with cataracts is at least similar to that in America and by combining the data in Figures 7-3 and 7-4, it is apparent that there cannot be many drivers with serious cataract involvement in the United States.

People undergoing cataract extractions presumably have been backed to the wall by failing vision and have been forced to have surgery performed. Presumably in the older age groups of sixty and beyond, job retention is not a factor but automobile driving might be. The person

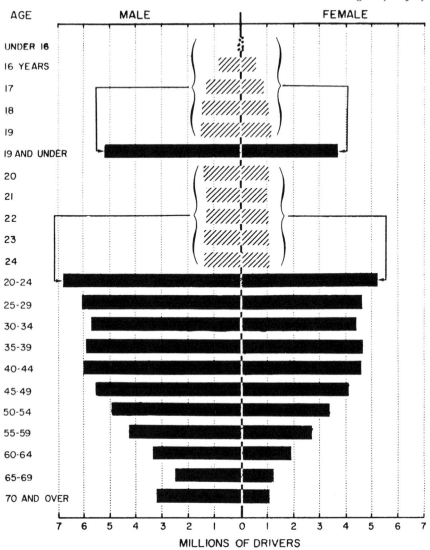

Figure 7-4. Breakdown of driving population in 1966 according to age and sex, from the U.S. Department of Transportation.

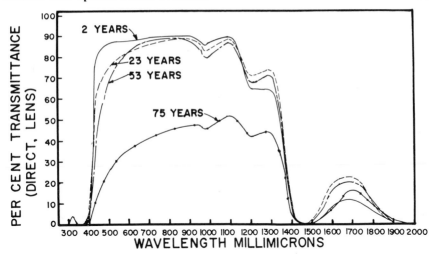

Figure 7-5. The influence of age and wavelength upon the transmission of the crystalline lens in the eye. The visible spectrum extends from 400 to 700 millimicrons. Comparison of curves two years and seventy-five years indicates that the older lens transmits only about 40 percent as much light as the younger lens. Since the lens is the element most affected by age in the eye, the age effect upon total ocular transmission can be assumed to be almost identical to these curves for the crystalline lens (Boettner and Wolter, 1962).

may have undergone surgery because he failed an eye test for renewing a driver's license or, in those states where vision tests are not given, the driver may have been badly shaken by discovering that driving on a busy highway at night with cataracts simply is not safe. Presumably they have had the surgery or have retired from trying to drive. Our data at this point cannot give us the answer.

In the early stages of diffuse cataracts visual acuity by day is often no different from normal, but at night the visual performance suffers enormously. In nuclear cataracts just the reverse is true. The greatest problem by day usually is the increased scattering of light by the cloudy lens and possible serious interference to vision when a nuclear or posterior capsular cataract is involved. Since night driving is accompanied by an enlarged pupil, the peripheral spokes in the lens of those over fifty-five years of age would be uncovered, so to speak, and stellate patterns of ocular scatter would result. It is of interest to note that increasing numbers of older people will not drive at night if they can avoid it even though they pass daytime vision tests with apparent ease.

Increased absorption of light in the eye with age is normal; see Figure 7-5 (Boettner and Wolter, 1962). By the time a cataract begins to interfere with measured acuity it has usually already become a serious hazard for nighttime driving. We find greater absorption and scatter of light with age, and irregularities in refraction, shifting cylinder powers and axes, and streaking of lights due to zonal defects in the lens. These defects may be due to variations in index and/or bulging of the lens contents between the Y sutures. The swollen lens thus resembles a bread roll, where the three segments of bread dough rise during baking to form three lobes attached by three straight lines. Of course the bread roll is a gross exaggeration, for it would require only a very slight localized swelling of the crystalline lens to cause the motorist great distress at night and to give the refractionist the problem of what would be the best lens prescription.

Since nighttime distress against headlight glare seems unrelated to ordinary daytime acuity test scores, some other test should be used to determine, if possible, how well the patient could be expected to perform at night. For this purpose the Night Vision Performance Tester described in Chapter 5 was developed.

Many researchers have recognized the interrelationship between contrast, luminance, and letter size in vision testing and have made equipment, gathered data, and advocated procedures for such testing. The effects of age have been studied and in some cases also the effects of refractive errors. The following are representative of such studies: Luckiesh, 1937, 1939, 1942, 1944; Fortuin, 1951; Guth, 1954, 1957; Allen and Lyle, 1963; Eastman et al, 1963; Richards, 1966; Forbes et al, 1967; Allen and Vos, 1967. All of the equipment in the above studies has shown that visual performance deteriorations with age are easily measured. These deteriorations are basically a reduction in contrast in the retinal image, a reduction in intensity of the retinal image, and possibly a reduction in physiological health of the retina and other nervous elements of vision.

Only a small percentage of people are continuing to drive who have cataract or other reduced vision problems in a sufficiently advanced stage to affect normal daytime clinical tests. Usually vision difficulties normally associated with old age are sufficient warning to most older people so that they do not attempt to drive, especially at night. However, for a large percentage of the population beyond forty-five years of age, the losses in performance are not forcefully felt and some test is needed to detect and determine the extent of their visual impairment, especially at night. At the beginning stages of significantly reduced performance, treatment may reverse the losses or delay their further development.

Early advice to the patient to improve his health by consulting his family physician can stop and may reverse the trend toward cataracts, even at an advanced age. Cataract development should never be assumed to be inevitable and untreatable, but rather to be a very sensitive sign of the patient's physical condition and to serve as a guide to the success or failure of efforts to improve his overall health. No single drug, nutrient, or vitamin known today seems to offer the specific treatment for clearing a cloudy lens. However, research into nutrition and other aspects of the cataract problem offers the hope of preventing and perhaps restoring the health of an early cataractous lens without the need for surgery.

Until such time as the answers about cataract development are known, a person is wise to maintain himself in the best possible health, which includes regular medical attention and supplementation of the daily diet with a well-balanced multiple vitamin and mineral formula, such as (or similar to) the one developed by Roger J. Williams (1962).

TABLE 7-4

Vitamins		*Minerals*		
Vitamin A	10,000 units	Calcium	300	mg.
Vitamin D	500 units	Phosphate	250	mg.
Ascorbic acid	100 mg.	Magnesium	100	mg.
Thiamin	2 mg.	Cobalt	0.1	mg.
Riboflavin	2 mg.	Copper	1	mg.
Pyridoxin	3 mg.	Iodine	0.1	mg.
Niacinamide		Iron	10	mg.
(or nicotinic acid)	20 mg.	Manganese	1	mg.
Pantothenate	20 mg.	Molybdenum	0.2	mg.
Vitamin B	5 mcg.	Zinc	5	mg.
Alpha tocopherol				
(Vitamin E.)	5 mg.			
Inositol	100 mg.			
Choline	100 mg.			

Such a formulation may be taken more than once a day with safety. Other authorities (Davis, 1965; Wohl and Goodhart, 1964) have different and apparently equally justifiable formulations; however, the minimum nutrients listed above and in these approximate proportions should give a guide as to the up-to-dateness of a formula being considered for purchase. The presence of respectable amounts of pantothenate and alpha tocopherol and the use of organic iron instead of the chloride or sulfate are clues to the newer formulations.

Past a certain point in development a cataract makes driving impossible at night. At a later stage driving by day becomes impossible as well. General daytime comfort and slightly improved performances can result from eye shades such as hats, sun visors, pinhole spectacles, and dark amber lenses. Such devices may increase somewhat the time that the developing cataract patient can continue to drive safely by increasing the optical contrast on the retina.

APHAKIA

Upon removal of the cloudy lens from the eye of the cataract patient, vision may be restored by spectacles or contact lenses. The best corrections with the least spatial distortions result with contact lenses. Because vision is nearly natural with contact lenses, the average aphakic will easily adapt to them. Provided the optical zone is large enough, the aphakic's vision while wearing the contact lens will be good both for day and night driving. In fact, the contact-lens-corrected aphakic will have excellent night vision because of the improvement in overall light transmission with crystalline lens removal. If retinal deteriorations have occurred with significant losses in the visual fields, visual acuity, or retinal sensitivity, driving a motor vehicle is inadvisable even with contact lenses.

Spectacle corrections for aphakia usually give good acuity; however, spatial distortions and blind areas at the margins of the lenses make driving hazardous and unwise where traffic is dense or swift. Aspheric spectacle lenses eliminate much of the spatial distortions and increase acuity in the marginal zones of the lenses, but they cannot relieve the blind zone at the edge of the plus lens (see Figure 7-6). However, because of the improved optical qualities of the aspherics, they can be prescribed in larger diameters, which moves the blind areas farther into the periphery and thus increases the visual field. Because of the overall spectacle magnification in aphakia, it is questionable whether even aspherics can make the spectacle correction for aphakia safe enough for driving a motor vehicle in high-density traffic.

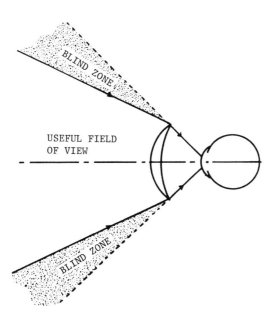

Figure 7-6. Blind zones created by a positive spectacle lens due to its magnifying properties.

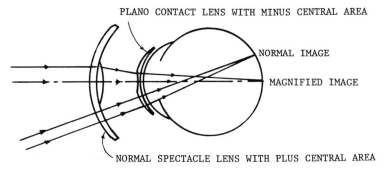

PLANO CONTACT LENS WITH MINUS CENTRAL AREA

NORMAL IMAGE

MAGNIFIED IMAGE

NORMAL SPECTACLE LENS WITH PLUS CENTRAL AREA

Figure 7-7. Telecon magnifying system. A contact lens with a small central area of high minus power is combined with a spectacle lens having a central zone of high plus power, thus constituting a Galilean telescope. The normally powered marginal regions of the contact lens and spectacle lens permit a wide field of view (Filderman, 1959).

LOW VISION

Because of losses in the peripheral field of view due to magnification of the central field and due to the supporting structures usually used, ordinary telescopic devices are not safe for driving even though they improve acuity. However, if the patient has normal peripheral fields and a telescopic unit is used that obstructs only a very small portion of the central field of view, it may be possible for the wearer to perform safely under favorable traffic conditions. There will always be a blind zone between the magnified portion of the visual field and the normal unmagnified part. The extent of this blind area depends upon the amount of magnification, the amount of the visual field magnified, and the pupil size. Figure 7-6 illustrates the optical problem involved, since aphakic correction lenses also magnify. The hardware for holding a telescopic unit before the eyes may or may not contribute to an increase in the extent of the blind area caused by the optical magnification.

The combination of contact lenses and spectacles to achieve telescopic effects usually provides a visual field with distortions and blind zones like those found in spectacle-corrected aphakia. A noteworthy exception is the Telecon lens system designed by Filderman (1959); see Figure 7-7. The Telecon system allows a magnified view straight ahead with normal vision laterally. The system works well on selected patients. If the patient can achieve acceptable central visual acuity, adapts to contact lenses and to the telescope system, he can be trained to drive safely.

Chapter 8: Visual Problems in
the Average Automobile

EYE POSITION ON THE HIGHWAY

THE TREND of automobile design is toward a lower silhouette. Few cars can provide an eye height of 48 inches even for above-average-height drivers. The low frontal area of an automobile is desirable for high speeds to reduce wind resistance, and the associated lowering of the center of gravity provides a greater resistance to roll-over. On the present highways and at the present highway speeds, however, it does not seem to be necessary to lower the vehicle profile for safety from roll-over, and therefore current trends appear to be almost entirely based upon styling and an effort to build a racing and sports-car image.

Practical considerations of passenger comfort and safety require that the size of the passenger automobile be about that of the New York Safety Sedan (Hildebrand and Wakeland, 1966), whose dimensions are as follows:

> Wheel base, 123 inches
> Tread, 62 inches
> Overall length, 220 inches
> Overall width, 80 inches
> Overall height loaded, 58 inches
> Loaded weight, 5100 pounds
> Engine, 260 h.p.

These dimensions provide room for an average family plus room for thick energy-absorbing doors, for interior padding, for energy-absorbing sheet-metal work in front and behind the passenger compartment, and for excellent roll-over protection. The eye height would be about 48 inches, depending on the driver and the seat adjustment. Very few American automobiles and practically none of the foreign automobiles are as large as the New York State Safety Sedan.

A little-realized complication of rakish styling is the loss of driver eye height above the road and the increased problem of lighting the roadway

100

as the vehicle height is lowered. The visual horizon depends upon eye height. The horizon of a six-foot man is about three miles away. When he sits in any of the low, fast, sporty American and European cars, he loses about a mile in seeing distance. For safety, an increase in speed requires a greater seeing range; hence the eye height in speedy sports cars should go up, not down. Distance judgments depend upon perspective clues, which are increased with increasing height. The time available for a motorist to recognize a hazard and react to it falls sharply as speed increases. Similarly, the ability to determine whether a developing situation is hazardous falls off as eye height is lowered. No one likes to be of short stature at a sports event or on a crowded sidewalk because he cannot see what is going on.

On level ground on the earth the effect upon the distance to the horizon of different eye heights is as follows:

TABLE 8-1

Eye Height in Feet	Miles to the Horizon
1	1.23
2	1.74
3	2.13
4	2.45
5	2.74
6	3.01
7	3.25
8	3.47
10	3.88

Headlighting also is critically dependent upon eye height. The higher the headlight the greater its potential range will be and the less its headlight aim will be disturbed by vehicle load and by a hilly road. On the other hand, the nearer it is to eye level, the greater the back scatter into the driver's eyes from his own headlights reflecting from atmospheric particles (dust, smoke, rain, snow, fog, and haze). Hence, the light must be both as far below the line of sight as possible and yet be as high above the roadway as possible.

The headlight system requires careful aiming to avoid glare in the eyes of the oncoming driver and yet provide illumination far ahead along the roadway. When the driver's eyes, the roadway, and the headlights are all very nearly in the same plane, as in sports car designs, glare cannot be divorced from lighting. Here again for optimum vision the eyes must be moved as high as possible above the plane of the lights, which must be as high as possible above the plane of the road.

If drivers' eyes are 42 inches above the pavement and headlights are 24 inches and aimed to light three hundred feet ahead, a change in a vehicle's load enough to tilt the front up 0.66 degree will place the headlight beam in the oncoming driver's eyes. This amounts to adding enough weight to the rear to lower it two inches in a fifteen-foot automobile. The lower the eye and light positions, the more critical is the aim and the more sensitive to load it becomes. An increase in the distance lighted on the highway makes the aim more critical. Since increasing the highway speed requires greater seeing distances which require greater headlight range, it is necessary, in order to keep reasonable headlight aim with varying load, that the lights and eye height be raised. High speed and low eye height cannot in any way be construed as a safe combination for the American highway.

For low automobiles it is essential that the aim of the headlights be independent of vehicle load or speed. This can be done by stabilizing the headlights themselves or by stabilizing the level of the vehicle so that headlights are properly aimed and the vehicle suspension operates at its optimum configuration. The driver's seat can easily be raised in future production, or a forward view telescope which effectively raises his eyes two or three feet can be installed. At any rate no significant improvement in vehicle headlighting can be made until headlight stabilization becomes standard on all American cars.

GLARE

Glare is a widely used word in the English language and is little understood. Everyone thinks he knows what glare is and how bad it can be. Everyone also thinks that sunglasses are to remove glare. But it is not this simple.

The *Dictionary of Visual Science* (Schapero et al., 1968) lists ten kinds of glare which may be condensed to three principal types: sensory overload, optical image degradation, and psychological annoyance.

Sensory overload begins to occur when the average luminance level exceeds 1,000 foot-lamberts. By 7,000 to 10,000 foot-lamberts, lacrimation and orbicularis spasms are normal symptoms, and visual performance falls rapidly. Optically, the image quality is the same or somewhat better at the higher luminances because of the smaller pupil.

Optical image degradation can occur via a uniform "film" of light scattered across the retina from a single bright glare source, such as every point of the white portion of this printed page, or from multiple glare sources, such as the multiple points of reflection on chromium automobile parts. Such a "veiling glare" effect serves to reduce the contrast in the optical image and hence to reduce visual performance—perhaps to zero. The image degradation is known to be worsened by pathology, refractive errors, and age; what may be a compensable glare to some may be incapacitating to others.

Psychological annoyance glare is also called *discomfort glare*. This is typified by the western sky in the late afternoon, which brightens as the sun comes down toward the horizon. A driver traveling west will ultimately find that the increasing sky brightness becomes uncomfortable. It is generally felt that discomfort glare has little relationship to veiling glare, although veiling glare also occurs in all such situations. Discomfort glare tolerance may be very low in certain refractive and pathological conditions.

Each of the foregoing three types of glare results in reduced visual performance. Only in the case of sensory overload can a sunglass be helpful, because for best vision the optimum scene luminance averages about 400 foot-lamberts. A demonstrable improvement in performance occurs if luminances of several thousand are reduced to that level.

Veiling glare B_v reduces performance proportionally according to the equation

$$B_v = \frac{K\, B_o}{\theta^n}$$

where B_o is the illuminance falling on the pupil from the glare source, θ is the distance of the glare source away from the line of sight in degrees, and constants K and n are approximately equal to 10 and 2 respectively. Differences in the formulas reported in the literature are largely due to age differences and other ocular conditions of the subjects and to the different methods of specifying the amount of glare light entering the eye.

The psychological or discomfort glare reduces performance three ways. Often there is an element of sensory overload when discomfort is

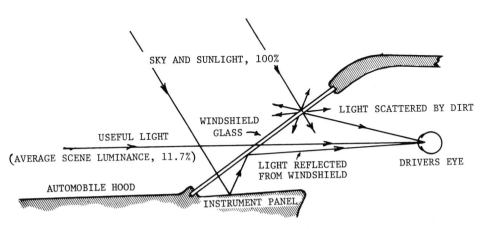

Figure 8-1. Sources of glare from the windshield and related structures. Note that the average useful light from the scene is 11.7 percent; thus dirt in full sunshine and/or the instrument panel top and windshield may easily direct enough light toward the eyes to be greater than the useful light.

experienced. The glare source scatters a veil of light throughout the eye and is of a significant amount when discomfort is experienced; hence deterioration in performance can be expected simply by sensory overload and image contrast reduction. The discomfort itself serves to reduce performance by providing a perceptual interference that may even reach the emotional level of anger or crying.

It is not well known that the driver's glare resistance is enhanced by a clean windshield, clean glasses, and an optimum correction for refractive errors and for vertical and lateral imbalances, as well as by the driver's momentary state of health and perceptual load. Recent experiments indicate that the effects of such factors as glare on performance, as measured in the laboratory will be about five times more detrimental on the highway in a nonexperimental situation. Either the perceptual load increases or attention to driving is reduced or both.

Glare light entering the driver's eyes comes from several sources, of which the windshield is one of the most important (Allen, Aug. 1969). Figure 8-1 shows the primary source of degrading or glare light caused by the windshield itself. The average scene reflectivity of 11.7 percent was determined by measurements as follows:

TABLE 8-2

Illuminance from Sky	*Illuminance from Earth*	*% Earth Reflectance*	*Earth Surface*
6900	1080	15.65	Concrete road
7000	880	12.57	Dirt
7100	500	7.04	Green field
7200	900	12.50	Blacktop
7200	1380	19.17	Gravel parking
7300	1040	14.25	Concrete
7400	950	12.84	Dirt
7700	380	4.93	Green field
7800	1280	16.41	Gravel road
8000	570	7.12	Blacktop
8150	830	10.18	City street
7850	680	8.66	City street
Av. 7466	872	11.7	Av. scene

To obtain the data in Table 8-2, the light meter was either directed toward the zenith, to obtain the illumination on a horizontal plane on the earth, or was directed horizontally, with a flat black shield lying horizontally on top of the light meter to block out all of the sky. Because the shield obstructed half of the receptive field of the photocell, its readings were doubled to get the values tabulated.

Figure 8-2 shows the other factors involved in automobile glare in addition to those of the windshield. Ray 1 is reflected from the hood

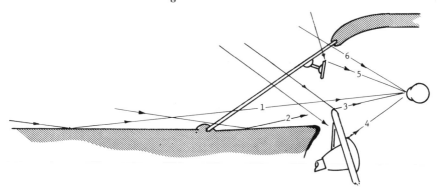

Figure 8-2. Nonwindshield sources of glare. The numbered rays are from glare sources as follows: (1) from the glossy hood paint, hood chromium, and fender chromium; (2) from the windshield trim, wiper hardware, speaker grille, and glossy dash panel top (especially pre-1967 automobiles); (3) glossy reflections from the rim of some steering wheels; (4) reflections from bright steering wheel hardware; (5) reflections from mirror hardware and chromed pillar post (windshield corner post); and (6) glare light directly from the sun and/or sky.

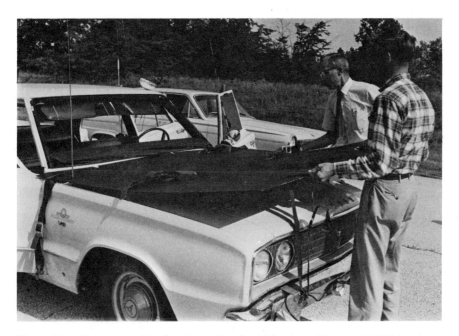

Figure 8-3. Test automobile for the study of vehicle glare. The windshield has been removed and the sun visors enlarged. The windows in the front doors have been covered with dark filter material, and the hood and dash panel top are being covered with a flat black material. Roadside targets were triggered by the vehicle 325 feet in advance and the reaction times needed for their detection by each of three observers in the front seat were recorded.

paint and hood or fender ornaments. Ray 2 is reflected from the dash panel, windshield chromium trim, and wiper hardware. Ray 3 is reflected from the steering wheel structure. Ray 4 is reflected from the chromium trim of the horn rim and steering wheel hub. Ray 5 is reflected from the mirror hardware, and Ray 6 is directly from the sun or from the open sky.

Figure 8-3 shows an instrumented vehicle with a detachable windshield used to evaluate the effect of glare encountered in typical daytime driving.

A study of forty-five drivers of all ages (Allen, Spring 1968) revealed that the most comfortable and efficient daytime driving occurred when all possible sources of glare had been removed. The windshield generally afforded the most predictable and important glare of all sources tested. At times sky glare, hood glare, and chromium glare were serious. When all sources gave maximum glare at the same time, the driver's performance was most adversely affected.

Tables 8-3 and 8-4 give the variations in sky luminance with the earth latitude, the time of year, and the time of day for a clear and for an overcast sky.

In Table 8-3 the values are taken so that the area around the sun and the sun itself are not measured. Note that on June 21 at 8 A.M. looking east and 4 P.M. looking west the sky is very bright and that in March and September at 10 A.M. and noon looking south the sky is very bright. In Table 8-4 when the sky is overcast, the luminances of the sky are more uniform so that directional effects are not significant. Because sky luminances are low, the illumination at ground level is likely to be much lower than when the sun is visible. Furthermore, the loss of shadows when the sky is overcast causes a loss of valuable target detail because of a loss of contrast which increases the visual handicap imposed by sky glare. Thus, overcast days are often more annoying to a motorist than a day of full sunshine. Evidence that this is so comes from subjective complaints and from the fact that motorists will turn on their headlights earlier at the end of an overcast day compared to a clear day.

TABLE 8-3
EQUIVALENT SKY LUMINANCE IN FOOT-LAMBERTS—CLEAR DAYS*

Latitude	December 21					March and September 21					June 21				
	8 AM	10AM	Noon	2 PM	4 PM	8 AM	10 AM	Noon	2 PM	4 PM	8 AM	10 AM	Noon	2 PM	4 PM
North															
30°N	450	600	600	600	450	700	1000	1050	1000	700	1550	1400	1000	1400	1550
34°N	350	550	550	550	350	800	800	900	800	800	1350	1400	950	1400	1350
38°N	300	550	550	550	300	750	800	900	800	750	1350	1300	950	1300	1350
42°N	250	500	500	500	250	700	750	800	750	700	1300	1300	950	1300	1300
46°N	150	450	500	450	150	700	750	750	750	700	1300	1250	950	1250	1300
South															
30°N	1100	1950	2250	1950	1100	1700	2300	2800	2300	1700	1200	1600	2400	1600	1200
34°N	1100	1900	2200	1900	1100	1700	2650	2900	2650	1700	1350	1650	2300	1650	1350
38°N	900	2300	2200	2300	900	1700	2700	2950	2700	1700	1350	1650	2300	1650	1350
42°N	600	2100	2150	2100	600	1700	2700	2450	2700	1700	1350	2000	2500	2000	1350
46°N	400	1900	2100	1900	400	1700	2700	2900	2710	1700	1350	2100	2700	2100	1350
East															
30°N	1550	1500	1000	700	400	2000	2500	1500	900	700	2800	2650	1400	1000	700
34°N	1350	1400	950	700	400	2400	2600	1600	950	650	2800	2700	1450	1000	700
38°N	1200	1300	900	650	350	2500	2600	1500	900	600	2800	2700	1400	1050	700
42°N	750	1200	850	600	250	2400	2400	1450	800	600	2900	2600	1400	1000	700
46°N	500	1100	800	500	150	2300	2100	1400	700	600	2850	2600	1400	1000	700
West															
30°N	400	700	1000	1500	1550	700	900	1500	2500	2000	700	1000	1440	2650	2800
34°N	400	700	950	1400	1350	650	900	1600	2600	2400	700	1000	1400	2700	2800
38°N	350	650	900	1300	1200	600	900	1500	2600	2500	700	1050	1400	2700	2800
42°N	250	600	850	1200	750	600	800	1450	2400	2400	700	1000	1400	2600	2900
46°N	150	500	800	1100	500	600	700	1400	2100	2300	700	1000	1400	2600	2850

* Average values, direct sunlight excluded.

TABLE 8-4

EQUIVALENT SKY LUMINANCE IN FOOT-LAMBERTS—
AVERAGE OVERCAST DAY

Latitude	8 AM 4 PM	9 AM 3 PM	10 AM 2 PM	11 AM 1 PM	Noon
December 21					
30°N	420	740	1020	1210	1270
32	350	700	960	1150	1200
34	320	650	910	1100	1140
36	260	600	840	1020	1070
38	230	550	790	940	1000
40	190	500	740	900	930
42	150	450	660	820	860
44	100	380	600	760	790
46	60	340	550	680	730
48	40	290	470	630	650
50	0	240	420	560	580
March 21 or September 21					
30°N	910	1320	1710	2010	2140
32	880	1290	1650	1940	2070
34	860	1250	1600	1870	1980
36	840	1220	1560	1800	1900
38	800	1200	1500	1740	1840
40	790	1140	1460	1670	1760
42	760	1120	1410	1600	1690
44	740	1080	1340	1540	1620
46	710	1030	1229	1470	1550
48	690	990	1240	1410	1480
50	650	940	1180	1330	1400
June 21					
30°N	1270	1730	2250		
32	1280	1730	2240		
34	1290	1730	2220		
36	1290	1730	2200	2960	
38	1290	1720	2160	2840	
40	1290	1700	2120	2650	3060
42	1300	1690	2080	2540	2860
44	1290	1670	2050	2430	2660
46	1290	1640	2010	2330	2520
48	1290	1620	1960	2250	2400
50	1260	1590	1900	2160	2280

To recapitulate, daytime glare is of multiple types and causation. Excessive overall illumination can be reduced with sunglasses, and visual performance will be increased. Specific glare objects that are excessively bright, such as chromium, hood paint, sky, and sun, adjacent to the normally bright visual task, cannot be toned down very much with sunglasses without a loss in visual performance. Sunglasses may reduce visual performance because they may reduce the useful light below optimum values, still leaving the proportion of glare to useful light unchanged;

and they also add a veiling glare of their own from dirt and surface re-flections. Discomfort glare is a function of total luminance, differential luminance, area, and distance from the visual task. Automobile glare is apt to approach the discomfort level even on overcast days in the daytime. For this type of discomfort, sunglasses may be helpful, but visual performance may not improve, especially on overcast days where overall luminances are already low.

Sky glare, road glare, water droplets, and dirt on the windshield all contribute significant amounts of glare, the total of which may be overpowering. Sun visors are a simple and effective means to control the sky glare. Some glare control comes from the color band at the top of the windshield. The windshield washer, when maintained, is an excellent means for reducing glare in bright sunshine by removing dust and dirt. The only beneficial defense the motorist has for glossy reflection glare from the roadway is a pair of polarizing sunglasses. For glossy reflections from the top of the dash panel, a piece of black velveteen cloth is superior to any surface finish yet devised.

Vehicular glare factors that can and must be controlled include the hood, which is usually shiny and may be of a light color; the chromium trim around windows, wipers, and steering wheel; interior window and door hardware; and the top of the dash panel. The 1967, 1968, and 1969 automobile production has greatly reduced the chromium glare which is found regularly in all automobiles of earlier manufacture. The hood still needs to be toned down in future production to a nonglossy, dark-colored surface. Some sport models now have black air scoops or a black pattern on the top of the hood.

The windshield continues to be a serious glare problem. Automobile stylists have not yet learned that the top of the dash panel is optically a part of the windshield and should be strictly off limits to decorators, painters, and artists who see no virtues in deep, rich black. In this case as in many others, doing it right will lend beauty and safety at the same time. It is commendable that high-gloss paints and vinyls on the dash panel top are no longer used, but many of the 1969 automobiles use colored vinyls that are not dull or dark enough. A fabriclike finish similar to black velveteen seems to offer the best solution to the dash-panel problem as now constituted.

The author's Dodge Polara has a modified dash panel covered with nylon flock imbedded in epoxy. The nylon fibers are electrostatically propelled onto the wet epoxy adhesive. Each nylon fiber stands at right angles to the surface to produce a durable equivalent of velveteen cloth. The surface is truly dead black, looks nice, and does not show dirt. This finish was also applied to a Coronet dash panel and hood. After twenty-four months the dash panel was still perfect, but the sun had bleached the nylon flock on the top of the hood. The process seems ideal for dash

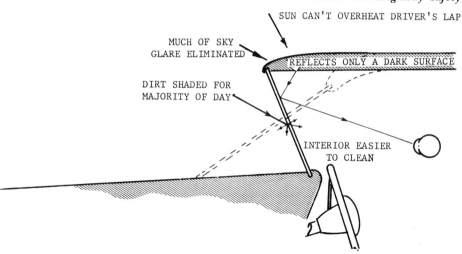

Figure 8-4. Characteristics of a windshield with a reverse tilt. Air cushion crash protection will keep passengers away from the windshield during a crash; hence the only design considerations are optical and aerodynamic. This design is optically superior.

panels and, if the material can be made sun resistant, its application to hoods is nothing short of a stylist's dream. No other feature on Indiana's research automobiles ever attracted so much attention as the black nylon flock on the hood of that white Coronet.

DIRT AND SCRATCHES ON THE WINDSHIELD

One solution to some of the more serious windshield problems is to tilt the windshield top forward, which is opposite to its present tilt (Figure 8-4). The glass would then reflect the shaded portions of the inside of the roof structure instead of the sun-illuminated dash-panel top. Such a tilt would also eliminate much of the problem of the dirty windshield by shading it in the daytime, since dirt per se is not as handicapping as the light reflected toward the driver from the dirt. The present windshield tilt exposes the dirt to full sunshine for over two thirds of the day.

The reverse tilt of the windshield would make it easy to get to the inside surface to keep it clean, an often neglected consideration. Outside cleaning would be somewhat more difficult, but the windshield would be inherently cleaner than it is now since it would not frost or collect dew at night as readily, or trap air-borne dust and dirt.

The only contraindication to such a design is aerodynamic. However, since vehicle stabilty at high speed is a serious problem, a lifting-air-foil upper contour of the automobile is not a desirable configuration. A number of land and water race drivers have died in vehicles that became air-borne without ailerons, rudder, or horizontal stabilizer, and an unknown number of passenger vehicle occupants have been injured or killed when they became air-borne when caught in a strong wind at high speed in a lightweight vehicle.

Since conventional automobile configurations do not assure ground hugging at high air speeds, a windshield redesign may be helpful as a lift spoiler needed to maintain vehicle stability. Lift spoilers are already in use on production automobiles as well as on racing cars.

Glare at night is mostly a problem of windshield dirt and scratches (see Figure 2–4). Allen (August 1969) has shown that the number of miles driven correlates with the number and severity of windshield scratches resulting from windshield wiper operation. It is estimated that at roughly 50,000 miles the windshield should be replaced to restore optimum vision at night against headlight glare. Some service station practices and some environmental factors, such as sandstorms and factory air pollutants, shorten the mileage over which a windshield can be safely used. A simple test for scratch deterioration can be made by observing from outside, through dark glasses, the reflection of the sun in the windshield. Focus your eye for the surface of the glass. A new glass will show a bright sun disc on a clear sky background. An older glass will show bright rings of scratches around the sun's image that extend out several inches from the edge of the solar image, masking the sky image. Driving an old car and a new car against headlights at night will illustrate the greater spread of headlight glare and the greater difficulty of seeing when looking through the older glass.

WINDSHIELD TINT

It is possible that the popular misconception that a tinted windshield reduces glare at night stems from comparing the old, scratched, nontinted windshield with the new unscratched tinted windshield at the time of buying a new car. When new untinted glass is compared with new tinted glass, however, the untinted glass gives a superior performance at night (Blackwell, 1954; Haber, 1955; McFarland and Domey, October 1958).

It is often argued that daytime comfort offered by the tinted windshield offsets the extra nighttime hazard. Such arguments do not hold up because (1) there is no proof that discomfort causes accidents, (2) there is evidence that comfort leads to inattention and—in the proper circumstances—to sleep, (3) the question of comfort is relative because tinted automobile glass removes not more than 50 percent of the direct solar heat energy and, (4) the nighttime hazard is greater than usually claimed because of the experimental method chosen to show that tinted windshields do not reduce seeing at night.

Many studies on tinted windshields have been conducted on the detectability of objects on the roadway as illuminated by low-beam headlights. Low-beam headlights are designed to give a sharp cutoff in light pattern on the roadway about 300 feet ahead, so that an object is not likely to be seen until it is close enough to enter the bright portion of the headlight pattern. At the forward edge of the headlight pattern the inverse square law does not hold, and a few feet of change in distance of the automobile from the object can change the illumination on that object at pavement level by a factor of 2 or more. Hence the reduction in seeing of a tinted windshield, which reduces light at the eye about 20 percent, compared to a clear windshield would be compensated for by allowing the object to move a few feet nearer into the headlight pattern. Thus, promoters of tinted windshields are able to say that only a 1 to 3 percent loss in seeing distance occurs due to a tinted windshield. Actually, if an object is not seen considerably prior to entering the low-beam headlight pattern it will probably be struck when traveling at 60 miles per hour. Windshield tint interferes most with the detection of unlighted vehicles or pedestrians on or near city streets, country roads, and highways. Obstacles in front and to the left will not come into the bright portion of the low-beam headlights pattern and will be rendered even less visible by a tinted windshield. As retinal luminance levels are reduced toward the absolute threshold, for example, by old age and windshield tint, the ability of the eye to discriminate subtle brightness differences falls off precipitously. At high levels a 1-percent brightness difference can be detected, whereas at the absolute threshold an object exhibiting a brightness difference from its background of 100 percent might not be detected.

A plate of glass loses light by surface reflection. Figure 8-5, Curve B, shows how the loss is dependent upon the angle of incidence of the light for a single surface. For two surfaces the loss is nearly doubled. Modern windshields are tilted to about 60 degrees from vertical, and it can be seen from figure 8-5 that a loss of about 20 percent due to reflection alone will occur with an untinted glass. Further inspection of Figure 8-5 reveals that the present windshield angle of American cars polarizes almost 100 percent of the light which it reflects. The amount reflected by a plate of glass at 60-degree incidence angle is about 20 percent; hence 80 percent is transmitted. This 80 percent is composed of 60 percent of the original amount of light which is unpolarized and 20 percent which is polarized. Hence, of the light transmitted, 20/80 or 25 percent is polarized.

Light reflected into the driver's eyes from the street, hood, and so on

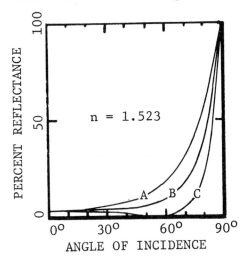

Figure 8-5. Effect of angle of incidence of light striking a single glass surface upon percent of light reflected. Curve B is the average reflectance of the ordinary and extraordinary rays striking the surface. On curve C the reflectance drops to zero near 55 degrees; thus only the A curve component of the light is reflected. In other words, the reflected light is completely polarized.

is partially polarized in the same plane as the light reflected from the windshield. In the daytime the angled windshield filters out most of the polarized component of specular glare from the pavement. However, by night, street lighting engineers *rely* on specular glare from the pavement to give efficient silhouette seeing with minimum wattage sources. The 60-degree angled windshield unfortunately removes a large portion of the polarized component of that light also.

The transmission curve of a tinted windshield is of interest, because it shows the relative efficiency of the windshield in removing heat radiation compared to visible light (see Figure 8-6). Solar energy is distributed about equally between visible and invisible radiation (see Figure 8-7); hence a windshield that absorbs all of the infrared and ultraviolet still transmits 50 percent of the heat energy. From Figure 8-7 it is apparent that the infrared and ultraviolet energy absorption is not perfect, nor is visible light transmission perfect. Figure 8-8 gives the ideal windshield tint, which would transmit all of the visible light available and remove all of the solar energy that does not contribute to vision. Only clear-white coated glass can come near the 100 percent transmission ideal in the visible portion, and there is no known way to retain the nearly 100 percent ideal in the visible portion and obtain complete absorption in the infrared and ultraviolet portions.

When windshield tint is present, angling the glass will increase the distance that the light has to travel to traverse the glass; hence the effect of the tint on the light will be increased. Figure 8-9 gives the results of measurements with a Pritchard Spectra Photometer on samples of clear

Vision and Highway Safety

and tinted windshield glass supplied by the Ford Motor Company. At 60 degrees away from the vertical, the clear windshield sample transmits 79 percent while the tinted windshield sample transmits 65 percent of the white light from a tungsten source. When the red filter in the photometer is used, the clear windshield transmits 75 percent, whereas the tinted windshield transmits only 49 percent of the red light from a tungsten source. The red filter in the Pritchard Spectra Photometer is tristimulus red and will not necessarily match the red filter in a given tail light or

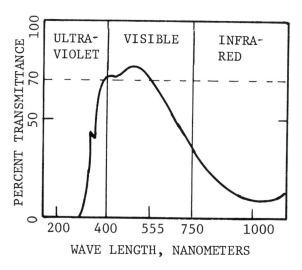

Figure 8-6. The transmission curve of a modern heat-absorbing automotive windshield (Whittemore, 1965). The bluish green color of this glass results from the lowered transmission of visible red light. Visible light lies between 400 and 750 nanometers (millimicrons).

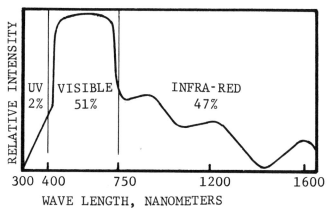

Figure 8-7. The relative intensity of solar radiation at each wavelength (Whittemore, 1965). The heat content of the visible portion of solar radiation is 51 percent, while for infrared (the "heat" radiation) only 47 percent is present.

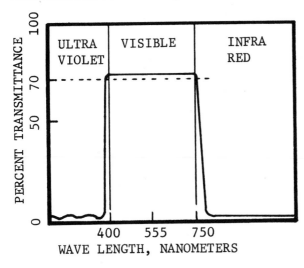

Figure 8-8. An "ideal" automative glass (Whittemore, 1965) would absorb all of the infrared and ultraviolet and only 70 percent across the spectrum of visible radiations. Such a glass would absorb about 64.3 percent of the solar energy. In practice only about 50 percent is absorbed. The arbitrary choice of 70-percent transmission across the visible spectrum is challenged in this book as hazardous at night and inadequate during the day.

stop signal. A deeper red—that is, one of longer wavelength composition —will be attenuated below the 49-percent measurement obtained because of the shape of the windshield transmission curve for red light (see Figure 8-6).

From these data one sees that the Society of Automotive Engineers' specification that a tinted windshield shall transmit not less than 70 percent visible light is misleading. The specification holds for vertical windshields and not for windshields in automobiles; and the specification ignores the selective absorption of tinted windshields for red light. If we are to hold to a 70-percent minimum allowable transmission, which most authorities have agreed to, it is apparent from Figure 8-9 that, even vertically, a tinted windshield cannot pass when tested for red light transmission! Furthermore, when installed in an automobile, the tinted windshield optimum sample tested indicates that only 65 percent overall transmission for visible light is possible. As matters stand now, it is not possible to meet the minimum SAE specification of 70 percent transmission with the present tinted glass. Hence probably all American automobiles with tinted windshields violate the intent of this specification!

A protanopic or protanomalous color-defective person is insensitive to red light (see Figure 8-10). A normal person looking through a tinted windshield has his color sensitivities disturbed somewhat similarly to a protanopic person. A person who is already insensitive to red, as are the protanopes and protanomals, will suffer even greater suppression of the red end of the spectrum through a tinted windshield (see Figure 8-10). The curves in Figure 8-10 are for a vertical windshield. To determine the effects of tilting the windshield, the data in Figure 8-9 should prove use-

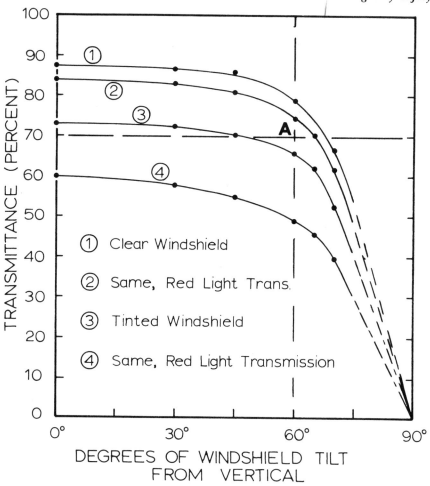

Figure 8-9. Plot of transmittances of a clear and a tinted (heat-absorbing) windshield for various tilt angles, and for red and white light transmission. Note that point A, the intersection between the tilt angle of 60 degrees and the Society of Automotive Engineers' lower limit of transmission, is above both the white light and red light transmission curves for a tinted windshield. These measurements were made on new one-foot-square samples supplied by an automobile manufacturer.

ful. The selectively greater loss of red light by a tinted windshield is evidence that it is hazardous in the daytime, since red signal and brake lights are not bright enough at best to be seen quickly in full daylight. The effect of the tint is to make the daylight relatively still brighter than the red signal light.

Another undesirable aspect of tinted window glass is that it reduces

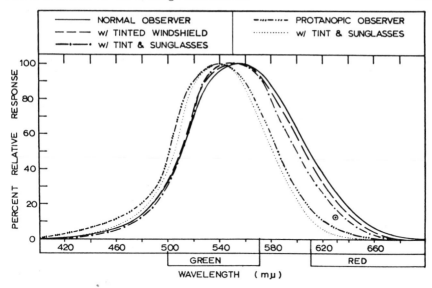

Figure 8-10. The effect of windshield tint and green sunglasses upon normal and protanopic (red-insensitive) luminosity curves when the windshield is vertical. Tilt of the
windshield to 60 degrees from the vertical will reduce the red end of the tinted windshield curves by about 26 percent (see Figure 8-9). The encircled dot at 630 mμ indicates
the effect of tilting a tinted windshield to 60 degrees when green sunglasses are worn by
a normal observer. This figure shows that if a protanopic driver wears green sunglasses
and peers through a tinted and tilted windshield it will be virtually impossible for him
to see any red light!

the chances of seeing the occupants of another automobile, thus further
reducing the chances for social interactions. Social interactions between
people is known to discourage antisocial behavior. Many feel that a person's bad driving manners would improve if other drivers could talk
about him or to him with a bull horn or a radio communications system between cars. Driving mistakes could be discussed and a sort of an
on-the-job training would result. Since we do not have this, the eye-to-eye
contact of drivers on occasion is very useful. Tinted window glass is often
so dense that one cannot be sure there are people in a car, let alone see
what their facial expressions are. Dark-skinned people are handicapped
in facial communication compared to fair-skinned people, because facial
expressions are washed out by simultaneous border contrasts when the
background objects are lighter in color. Hence facial features and expressions cannot be fully appreciated.

Another adverse feature of tinted automobile glass is the inability to
see through two or more cars if their windows are tinted. A driver attempting to pass must therefore practice the dangerous peek-a-boo operation of pulling far enough to the left to see around. In regard to tilt

angle, heat-absorbing efficiency goes down the more nearly the glass faces the sun; at the same time the amount of glare light reflected from the sky toward other drivers increases. This increased sky or sun reflection from the windshield tends to obscure the view of the people in the car, accentuating the obscuration due to tint.

DISTORTIONS

Distortions exist either as small or major surface defects in front, rear, and side windows. Small surface defects, or orange-peel-like irregularities, show up as blurred vision, while major surface defects produce gross displacements and distortions of objects from their true location and shape. Larger waves and ripples in the glass are mainly caused by variations in thickness; they produce major distorting effects of size and position of objects seen through the glass. Microscopic defects, such as inadequate polish or metallic deposits in the case of float glass, cause light scatter and blurred vision.

A survey in December 1967 of autos in the 1968 Indianapolis Auto Show showed startlingly poor windshield quality. When checked for orange-peel texture, four Lincolns, 100 percent, were rated as reject, and three or four Chryslers were reject (Cadillac was not evaluated). The company scores were as follows: General Motors, three good, twelve average, and one (Toronado) reject; Chrysler, three good, thirteen average, and three reject; Ford, two good, two average, and four reject. A midyear check of 1969 automobiles found windshields remarkably improved. The new ratings showed Ford's window glass best, with that of Chrysler and General Motors about the same, good, but not quite as good as Ford.

The major surface defects are most serious when trying to see through the vehicle ahead. The combination of rear window and front window distortions may be considerably greater than the simple sum of the two distortions; hence rear window distortions as well as windshield distortions need to be minimized. Quality control of gross distortions is improving; most 1969 and 1970 cars have reasonably good see-through ability where the size and slant of the rear window allow. See-through distortions that raise the scene or minify it make approaching cars seem farther away. Those that confuse the scene by multiple small irregularities may obscure the presence of an approaching car or force the following driver to move to the left to see around the lead car. Experience indicates that most motorists are not content to follow a vehicle they cannot see through.

Major distortions in the windshield itself are serious and are encountered to some degree among each manufacturer's products. Variations in sheet glass production, in heat forming, in lamination procedures, and in materials combine to produce one windshield of reject quality while the next one will be acceptable. Whether the rejects are rejected is a matter of inspector alertness and company quality control standards. The author has seen windshields in showroom display automobiles with ripples, swirls, "orange peel," haze, and even a dimple directly in the forward view of the driver. Both salesmen and managers alike looked on unbelievingly when these defects were pointed out. Obviously the public and the company men in the field were not able in the past to recognize these flaws.

Major distortions near the right side of the windshield are still seen and, in effect, enlarge the corner post obstruction. The method of manufacture determines in good part how much distortion there will be. When one is entering a roadway, vehicles approaching from the right and viewed through even slight distortion can be misjudged both as to speed and distance, and the distortion may cause driver behavior similar to that of not having seen the approaching vehicle at all. Major distortions near the straight-ahead position can cause double images, eye fatigue, headache, and nausea. These symptoms may or may not interfere with driving efficiency, depending upon the person and the severity of the distortion. Distortions near the left corner post are especially hazardous when turning left and in detecting pedestrian and vehicle traffic approaching from the left. In effect the left corner post is enlarged by glass distortions.

Side-window gross distortions do not seem particularly hazardous to the driving operation. However, these distortions do impair see-through ability by other drivers in numerous instances, and generally a car is labeled as low quality if obvious distortions are present. It is probable that children and other passengers are more likely to have car sickness when side and rear windows are distorted.

Often we hear that the curved windshield is the cause of all manner of distortions and that a flat windshield would be better. Actually a curved windshield with the eye at the center of curvature is the more ideal arrangement (see Figure 8-11). Viewing through a flat plate of glass at an oblique angle reduces transmission and exaggerates any irregularities in the surface and optical media as well as creating an astigmatic-like blur of the object viewed. The gentle curvature of the modern windshield is a reasonable compromise. However, the slope angle of 60 degrees backward tilt away from the vertical is a major source of light loss, dirt, internal reflections, glare, heat build-up, and optical distortions and is *not* ideal for any *optical* purpose.

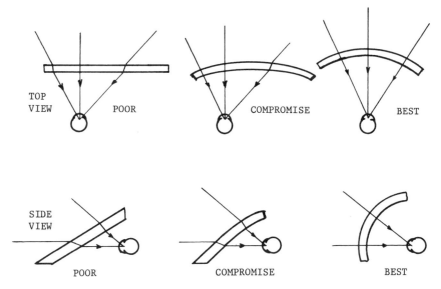

Figure 8-11. Schematic diagram of some possible windshield designs. In general a concentric design would give zero distortion and negligible refractive power if the thickness were small.

OBSTRUCTIONS AND THE REAR-VIEW MIRROR

The largest single obstruction in the driver's visual field is usually the inside rear-view mirror. The placement of this mirror seems not to be determined by the eye height of the 95th-percentile driver but by the position of the rear window, which seems to obey no rules of visual design. As a result, most hard tops and almost all sedans have a serious obstruction due to the low position of the rear-view mirror. A survey of 1960–1962 automobiles (Allen, December 1962) showed that the rear-view mirror occupied 14 to 18 degrees of the field of view and was between 32 to 53 degrees to the right side of straight ahead. In comparison the left windshield corner post varied beween 5 and 17 degrees in lateral dimension and was located between 10 and 26 degrees to the left of straight ahead of the driver's eyes. The right windshield corner post was about 5 degrees in thickness and was about 75 degrees away from straight ahead. The general trend in 1969 toward racy styling has made these visual obstructions worse. In addition, designers have cramped the driver and passengers and markedly increased the obstructions caused by the rear roof line, the rear quarter panels, and the front roof line.

The outside rear-view mirror is improperly located on some vehicles. Federal standards in 1967 first required that outside rear-view mirrors be placed on all automobiles. The intent of this standard was that the required outside rear-view mirror should be as large and as far forward as possible. However, on some 1968 and 1969 cars, one must turn his head and eyes almost 90 degrees to the left and downward to see in the mirror. (Ample space and window coverage is provided in most cases forward of the factory installed position, sometimes as much as a foot farther forward.) While looking in such mirrors the driver cannot see with his peripheral vision any of the roadway ahead; hence the placement of such outside mirrors can be expected to cause accidents. Notable improvement in outside mirror placement has occurred in some 1969 cars having one-piece door glass without the vent wing.

A properly designed periscopic rear-view mirror might eliminate the need for the outside mirror as we know it today. Periscopic and other exotic rear-view mirror designs have been around for several decades. They range from the simple convex single mirror through complex lens-reflector designs using astigmatic elements. Experimental systems include television displays, radar detectors, and laser ranging devices. Systems which offer the most information in a practical and relatively inexpensive assembly are those based upon flat mirrors arranged several different ways.

Flat mirror systems are more desirable than other systems because they are inexpensive; they are not subject to distortion; they give no inherent enlargement or reduction in the image viewed, hence space perception is normal; they permit a wide range of head and eye movements; and ideally arranged, they permit rearward view by simply looking upward slightly, thus not interfering seriously with forward vision.

All other systems suffer from serious disadvantages. For example, the television display of rearward scenery must of necessity be confined to a small area on the dash or elsewhere. This means that size and distance information are grossly distorted; resolution is reduced by the amount of the size reduction needed to get a large field of view; being a near task, the driver must accommodate before meaning can be gained from the miniature display; and those drivers over forty-five years of age may not be able to focus on the display due to presbyopia. This is not to say it cannot be done, but at present a television rear-view display loses more than it gains, and training is needed to get the most out of what is left. It is simply not possible to interpret accurately what is "out there" by what you see in that little window which is obviously close by. Almost the same problems exist with the convex rear-view mirror which is commonly placed adjacent to a flat mirror to help compensate for its limitations.

Principles to be observed in the construction of periscopic systems with flat mirrors are as follows: (a) an even number of reflections is needed for forward vision, (b) an odd number of reflections is needed for

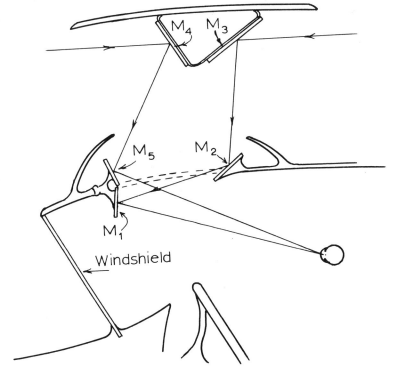

Figure 8-12. Periscopic combination forward and rear-view mirror systems for simultaneous viewing from one eye position.

        M_1 Mirror, adjustable about horizontal axis, rear view
        M_2 Mirror, fixed, rear view
        M_3 Mirror, fixed, rear view
        M_4 Mirror, fixed, forward view
        M_5 Mirror, adjustable, forward view

rearward vision, (c) the system should be as short as possible from the eye to the exit aperture to ensure the largest field of view, (d) filters should be avoided and as few optical elements used as possible because light losses are related to the number of elements, (e) direct sun on any component and sky glare in the field of view should be avoided, and (f) the final mirror should be placed directly ahead and above the line of sight of the driver to avoid obstructions in the field of view.

Rearward and forward periscopic vision might benefit from a windshield tilted forward at the top because it would provide the extra room needed for the optics. Figures 8-12 and 8-13 give the essentials of two designs of periscopes for automobile use. These combine forward and rear-

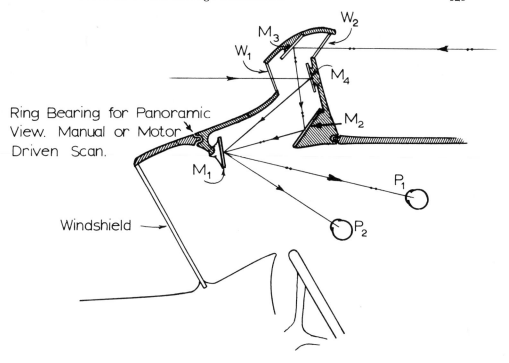

Figure 8-13. Periscopic combination forward and rear-view mirror systems requiring two-position viewing. The normal eye position, P_1, would permit a periscopic rearward view, whereas movement of the head forward to P_2 would provide a periscopic forward view. Mirror M_1 is adjustable to allow for driver height. Fixed mirrors M_2 and M_3 provide a rearward view through window W_2, while fixed Mirror M_4 provides a forward view through Window W_1.

ward visibility, with selection of view being based upon a simple movement of the eyes or movement of the head to look forward. The intentional movement forward to gain a forward view would guard against becoming confused as to which scene was being looked at.

INSTRUMENT PANEL VISIBILITY

The major factors contributing to the speed and accuracy of instrument panel readability in the daytime are the illumination on the display compared to the illumination on the road, the size of the numerals or letters, the contrast of the numerals or letters with their background, the accommodative ability of the eyes of the driver, and the placement of the seat and the steering wheel.

The speed of recognition of the critical dial or gauge is increased with larger sizes, greater illumination, greater contrast, and a younger driver who can focus his eyes more quickly.

A study on 1960, 1961, and 1962 automobiles (Allen, February 1963) showed that the average eye-to-dash-panel distance was 72 cm. in fifty-six automobiles with the seat in the position in which it was found when the vehicle was first encountered for testing. The height of each of the numbers on the speedometer averaged 1 degree 16 minutes, and each odometer numeral averaged 20 minutes in height. At that time the illumination on the dash panel ranged from 46 to 1,640 foot-candles. The average scene luminance in the first case was 634 and in the second case 852 foot-candles.

Improvements have been made in dash panel design in general, but some 1969 automobiles still have small dials and numerals and/or they are deeply recessed so that illumination is a problem. An outstanding speedometer display has been used in many models in which the numerals are large, widely spaced, and far away from the driver's eyes for easy and quick recognition. Other manufacturers have used large displays from time to time, but instrument panel design cannot be said to be at all standardized as of this writing. The designs range from the most fully instrumented down to the absence of all instruments except the speedometer and gas gauge. Instrument clustering cannot be standardized when instruments themselves have not been standardized. Instrument dial size depends upon the space available in a particular model and upon esthetics as much as upon visual criteria of speed of readability.

A study (Allen, October 1964) was made on fifty new 1963 automobiles in dealer stocks of the time required to look from the sun-lighted exterior scene to the dash panel and recognize a speedometer numeral. The two observers were seventeen years of age and pretrained for five days to build up their reaction time skills. The average time of these practiced subjects to clear the dash panel without sunglasses was 0.717 seconds, while the same task required 0.781 seconds with fit-over sunglasses. In addition to this first recognition time a driver would still have to search until he found the speedometer needle or other gauge of importance. Following this he must return his eyes to the outside scene. It may be conservatively estimated that a normal driver of thirty-five to forty years of age will require at least two seconds to inspect the average dash panel and return his gaze to the highway. Some panels and some conditions would greatly lengthen this time.

A pair of glasses tinted in the upper and clear in the lower portions, combined with a properly powered bifocal for older drivers, makes a significant improvement in the speed of inspecting the dash panel and returning vision to the highway.

Dash-panel visibility at night depends upon the same factors as for daytime visibility except that panel lighting is supplied artificially. The best illuminant depends upon the nature of the driver's refractive error. A hyperope and an emmetrope would see best at near with blue-green or blue light, whereas a myope or a bifocal wearer might see better with red light because of the 1.80 diopters of chromatic aberration error existing in the human eye. At night the loss of surround lighting can contribute to disorientation, double vision, and drowsiness. This effect can be reduced by brightening up the instrument panel illumination and, if needed, by turning on the interior ceiling light.

HEADLIGHTS

AIM

Improper headlight aim because of lamp replacement, bent fenders, broken or sagging springs, or unusual vehicle load is a major cause of glare at night, but for a reason different from what most people think. Improper headlight aim modifies the illumination pattern in front of the automobile to less than optimum. This means that for a low beam aimed too low, the seeing distance is reduced, though the brightness of the illuminated road surface is higher than normal. If the low beam is aimed too high, a greater seeing range is provided, but the illumination on the pavement needed for vehicle guidance will be lowered. Within limits, in either case, there is not much difference in glare to oncoming motorists on a straight highway because of the cutoff at the left of the low beam pattern that is characteristic of American headlights. However the loss in headlighting range with a beam that is too low, and the loss in pavement illumination when the beam is too high, renders the driver with poorly aimed headlights more susceptible to ordinary glare light from other cars.

Glare at night is more a matter of the difference in luminance levels between the glare source and the visual task than of the intensity of the glare source alone.

Anything which destroys the headlight aim or distribution built into the lamp will increase glare at night. Although faulty headlight aim as just indicated is an important factor, dirt and scratches on the headlight lens produce equally important degradations in headlight efficiency. The light that is diverted from the roadway is scattered in part toward the oncoming driver's eyes. At the same time the losses of light on the roadway make oncoming headlights appear brighter or more glaring.

Gadgets sold to be attached to headlights are almost always harmful. For example, yellow filters absorb blue light as well as lose about 8 percent of the white light by reflection. "Sleepy-eye" chromium covers used over the top half of the head lamp lens are especially detrimental since they destroy the headlight pattern, thereby increasing the glare into oncoming drivers' eyes and reducing the useful illumination. Improving light output pattern and increasing headlight power gradually over a period of years should be encouraged—preferably paced by the automobile and lamp manufacturers. The importance of headlight aim and pattern should be emphasized in new car literature and automotive magazines, with cautions clearly stated as to the hazards of covering the head lamp with anything, including dirt.

TABLE 8-5
HISTORY OF AUTOMOBILE HEADLIGHTS

Years	Type of Lamp	Upper Beam	Lower Beam
1902–1906	Oil	—	—
1906–1912	Acetylene	—	—
1912–1915	Tungsten in vacuum	—	—
1915–1924	Lenses introduced; tungsten gas filled	—	—
1924–1928	Two filaments, upper and lower beam	300 feet	80 feet
1928–1934	Fixed focus	340 feet	130 feet
1934–1939	Prefocused flanged bulbs	390 feet	175 feet
1939–1955	7″ sealed beam dual filament	400 feet	210 feet
1955	Improved 7″ sealed beam with filament cap; better in fog, rain	420 feet	280 feet
1958	5¾″ dual sealed beam, designed for optimum performance on both high and low beams.	430 feet	300 feet
1959	7″ Type 2 sealed beam, improved low beam	400 feet	300 feet
1969	Quartz halogen high-intensity sharp cut-off meeting light, Chrysler Corporation's Super-Lite	—	400 feet

Many automobiles are so sensitive to load that two male adults in the rear seat are enough to require re-aiming of the headlights. In 1969, manufacturers made it possible to reach headlight adjustment screws without removing chromium trim. This was an important improvement because it speeds headlight adjustments and permits a motorist to adjust his head lamps a few degrees to correct for an overload of his vehicle.

The next step is to provide adjustment with a thumb screw and a dial for setting the lights to match the load. The ideal is a load-stabilized vehicle that maintains the same level whether loaded or empty. As soon as this becomes standard, significant increase in headlight candle power can be made.

FILAMENT SHIELDS

High-beam head lamps used in four headlight arrays do not have filament shields to prevent upward scatter into rain, snow, and fog, whereas low beams do. These shields are the result of an invention by Orville Stamm who personally for seventeen years extolled their virtues and attempted to interest the automobile industry and the several large manufacturers of lamps. In 1955, after his patent had expired, the lamp manufacturers began to advertise an improved fog-penetrating head lamp incorporating a shield. Certainly, the United States Patent Office protects the inventor, but it has, on occasions such as this, deprived the public of safety advancements for seventeen years while the inventor wastes his time, effort, and money trying to find a manufacturer willing to pay a royalty on a patent.

SLEEPY-EYE SHIELDS

On the other hand, headlight sleepy-eye shields (see Figure 8-14), used by the younger set, are rightfully not sold by the automobile manufacturers. While manufacturers have not adopted or endorsed them, neither have they strongly opposed them—or dozens of other "sucker trade" accessory items offered for sale on the "after market." The sleepy-eye shield increases glare, reduces roadway illumination, and destroys the Society of Automotive Engineers' specified headlight beam pattern (Allen, January 1967). It is especially poor in snow, rain, and fog because of increased light randomly distributed. The results of the study on these shields were sent to the Federal Trade Commission. As of this writing, the devices are still being sold.

DISAPPEARING HEADLIGHTS

Headlights that are covered when not in operation are a true salesman's gimmick which has hazardous complications. Being mechanical, they are subject to failure and wearing out. Some lamps remain fixed and their covers open and close; others move with the covers and are not properly aimed until the operation cycle is completed. Thus, interferences with aim as well as the chances for mechanical failure exist.

Complications occur even in properly operating disappearing head lamps. They are exposed only when hot, and road splatter dries on them. When the lamps are cool and could be rain washed or noticed by the station attendant and washed, they are covered. The build-up of dirt destroys the headlight distribution pattern and attenuates the light, thereby increasing the glare to oncoming motorists and effectively increasing the glare of oncoming headlights by reducing the light on the pavement.

A second complication of disappearing headlights is the inability to use them in the daytime to signal an oncoming driver. The lights are allowed up to three seconds to go into full operation (U.S. Department of Transportation, 1968). A time interval of two seconds will allow two automobiles each approaching at 60 miles per hour to come 352 feet closer to one another; hence disappearing headlights are as useless in the daytime as the horn for warning oncoming drivers on the highway.

There appears to be no justification for covering the headlights. We have few gravel roads and we are not a nation of race drivers. The only advantage seems to be styling. Styling also can be hazardous because the front and rear of the automobile now look almost identical when the headlights are covered. The disappearing headlight was put on the market at a time when great resistance was shown by the manufacturers to such things as energy-absorbing steering columns and dual brakes. The development cost for disappearing headlight designs probably equaled or exceeded the cost of each of the safety features that the industry was required to install and to which they objected so loudly, at least in the beginning.

It is now clear that in the near future all automobiles will wear lights in the daytime which will come on as soon as the engine is started. Low-beam headlights are reasonably well suited for front-of-the-car running lights for daytime use and are recommended for that purpose

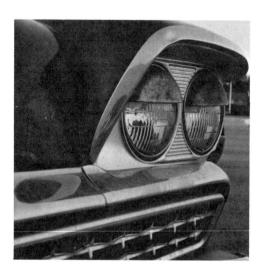

Figure 8-14. Sleepy-eye shields. According to the usual description on the carton, shields like this reduce glare for oncoming drivers and increase vision for the owner. It may be recommended that high beams could be used at all times with such shields in place. One can't help thinking that if covering 40 percent of a headlight is so beneficial, think how beneficial it would be if 100 percent of the headlight were covered!

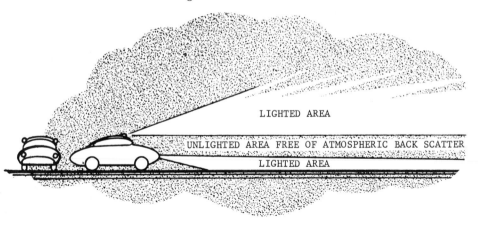

Figure 8-15. Recommended vehicle lighting for forward vision. Regular headlights would be designed to have a limited upward component to prevent lighting particulate matter in the atmosphere before the driver's eyes. To permit reading freeway signs and stop signs, which are usually above eye level, the smaller top-mounted lights would be used.

(Allen, September 1965). Better side and rear lighting will need to be developed for daytime use. It is hoped that disappearing headlights will themselves disappear as unnecessary cost items and that it will not be necessary to require installation of another running light to be on at all times, day or night, when the vehicle engine is operating.

All-weather Headlighting System

An ideal all-weather system installed in self-leveling automobiles would be one that puts no light at all into a zone between three and five feet above the road (see Figure 8-15). Thus there would be very little back scatter from fog, rain, or snow and the seeing range would therefore be increased. Sharp-cutoff head lamps are already available, as demonstrated by Chrysler with their Sylvania-manufactured Super Lite. Since such a headlight cannot light overhead signs or signs along the roadside without crossing the zone between three and five feet above the pavement, headlights mounted above eye level are needed. These would be aimed so that no light drops below five feet. Because they would be nearer to the driver's eyes than are the conventional headlights, they could be somewhat less powerful and still provide adequate illumination for seeing overhead retroreflectorized signs. In addition, such roof-mounted headlights, one at each side, would shape-code the front of the automobile with a rectangular pattern of white lights which could not be confused with present tail light patterns or with the compatible proposed future tail lighting system described in the next section.

SIGNAL VISIBILITY

FRONT SIGNALS

American automobiles suffer from a poorly designed signal system. For instance, front turn signals are not visible to adjacent cars in multilane traffic because they are placed too low and are aimed only in the forward direction. Some models are not even visible to a pedestrian standing within a car length from the front of the car unless he squats down. Except for being in a desirably shaded location, all other evidence indicates that turn signals should be raised to the top of the fender. This would permit visibility of the signal from all angles, including the side and rear. American production has incorporated the less desirable European system of using the parking light in front when the headlights are on low beam. This provides the identification clue that may be needed when one of the headlights burns out; however, actual highway counts involving 9,000 vehicles showed that only about one car in 500 had but a single headlight in operation. The undesirable aspect of having the parking lights on in traffic is that amber now becomes a front running light which is on all the time that the headlights are on low beam. In addition, the regular use of parking lights reduces the signal value of the turn signal, which usually has its filament within the same bulb. The use of amber on the front overlaps the currently permitted amber for rear presence, turn, and brake lighting as used on some foreign automobiles. Among color-defective as well as normal people, amber is often confused with red (Heath and Schmidt, 1959). Of the signal colors red, green, and yellow (or amber), the yellow is the weakest and produces the most mistakes in color recognition; it is sometimes called white, red, or even green. In the daytime, body styling confuses the front and rear appearance of automobiles. The confusion is reinforced by amber lighting on the front. At night under certain conditions, especially when only the parking lights are on, the use of amber on the front also confuses the front and rear of an automobile.

REAR SIGNALS

COLOR. Rear-end lighting suffers important deficiencies. Two percent of male drivers have a sensitivity to red light of about one fifth or less (depending upon the wavelength composition of the red light) compared to a color-normal individual. Furthermore, tinted windshields, which are estimated to have been installed in well over half of American automobiles, further reduce the transmission of red light compared to white or green light. To correct for these losses, tail lights would need to be five times brighter or of a color other than red. The sensitivity to green is not adversely affected by any of the common color vision defects or space perception aberrations (Allen, December 1964); hence its use for a rear running light is highly recommended.

There is an opposing argument that since about 5 percent of the male population are deuteranopes or deuteranomals who confuse green with white, the difference between the front and rear ends of an automobile is lost for them if green tail lights are used. The answer to the following question is the only answer of consequence to this argument: Would you prefer, while in a fog or under other adverse circumstances, to be a deuteranope encountering two lights that you can't be sure are green or white, or to be a protanope encountering a similar situation and vehicle whose two red tail lights you cannot see at all? The inability to see a light and hence not to know that a hazard exists seems to be a far more dangerous traffic handicap than is the confusion as to whether you are looking at the front or the back end of a hazard. Actually, since tail lighting is so much less intense than the white headlights, the distinction between front and rear is easily made on the basis of intensity, just as millions of decisions about the difference between tail and brake lights are made every day.

POSITION. For an open highway with low traffic density, tail lights and brake lights need to be low for maximum appearance of nearness. When traffic becomes heavy, a high-position for tail lights and brake lights at the roof line of a passenger car is needed to permit them to be seen through other cars and to reduce the chances of a multiple rear-end collision.

When automobiles are traveling close behind one another on a straight, level stretch of roadway, a slight change in velocity of the lead car can cause a touch of the brake for the second and third cars, a panic braking for the fourth and fifth, and a rear-end collision for most of the rest. Thus is born the spectacular freeway pile-up. If the second driver could signal the fifth driver behind him that he had touched his brake, that driver would know of the hazard just as soon as the drivers who are nearer. By thus increasing the range of brake lights by five cars, the first rear-end accident would not occur until the twenty-fifth car back instead of the fifth, a saving of twenty cars! Furthermore, the severity of the collisions that did occur would not peak as quickly, and more vehicles would escape with light damage.

In a study (Allen et al., February 1967) using auxiliary tail lights mounted near the top of the windows of a station wagon, the signal was found to penetrate to at least the third driver behind the lead car without time attenuation, whereas ordinary tail lights required that each driver see the brake light ahead of him and put on his brakes to signal the man behind him to put on his brakes.

Figures 8-16 and 8-17 show the improvements in performance ob-

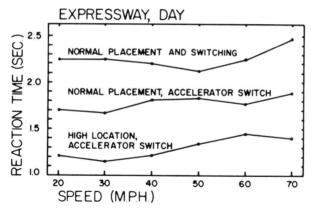

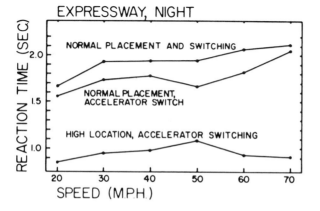

Figure 8-16. Drivers' reaction times at various speeds on the daytime expressway following test vehicles with two rear lighting arrangements and with brake and accelerator switching.

Figure 8-17. Same as Figure 8-16 except data taken at night.

tained in following behavior when the tail lights were raised and when a switch was put on the accelerator which lighted the tail lights before the foot could get to the brake pedal. It is apparent that performance is best when the driver can see through the car ahead. It is also improved by accelerator switching of the brake light. In this experiment three drivers and a timer operator had to react when the lead vehicle applied its brakes. By subtracting a simple reaction time of 0.2 second for the timer operator, the average driver reaction time using the stock brakes was 0.58 second. With the high-positioned accelerator-switched brake light system, the individual driver reaction time averaged 0.25 second. In other words, high placement of brake lights can transmit information to a train of *closely following* drivers much quicker than the stock brake lights can.

While there is a clear superiority of placing the brake light at eye level when cars are traveling close together, as on freeways, it is not proper to assume that the present tail lights should be replaced with roof-mounted lights. The tail light function is best located below eye

level, to localize the position of the vehicle with respect to the driver's horizon. The high-position brake light should be in addition to the stock
brake lights and not a substitute for them. Since roof heights vary among
vehicles, the high signal light placement should be at a standardized
height above the pavement; for example, 60 inches.

In keeping with space perception cues it is desirable to make the car
ahead of you appear as close as possible. This is done by lowering the
regular tail (presence) lights and by increasing their luminance, their size,
and their lateral separation. When brakes are applied it is desirable to increase still more the apparent nearness of the stopping vehicle. This is
done by increasing the spacing and the intensity and by reducing the
height of the brake lights compared to the tail lights. Thus, brake lights
should be outside of the tail lights and should be larger, brighter, and
lower. Figure 8-18 shows the brake lights at the same level as the presence lights, because the presence lights have been placed as low as prac-
ticable to enhance their location-fixing value.

Shape Coding. As indicated in the preceding section, higher placed
lights also must be added to help prevent freeway collisions. These are in
effect high-placed repeater lights, but they could serve another most valuable function. They would increase the apparent size of the rear end of a
vehicle and would provide the means for effective shape coding (see Figure 8-18). For example, a midline green light at the top of a passenger
automobile would form the apex of a green triangle when green tail
lights were used, while a red brake light at each outer edge of the top,
combined with the regular brake lights, would complete a red square of
light for a brake signal (see Figure 8-18). The separate turn signal lamp
in the conventional lower location should be supplemented by a repeater
lamp adjacent to the high-mounted red brake light repeater position, and
it should also be green (Marsh, 1967).

By making the red brake lights include a good deal of yellow, they
would be seen by protanopic color defectives. The approximately rectangular shape would identify them as stop lights even if the observer were
color defective. The triangular rear green lights would not be confused
with the front of a vehicle, even if the driver saw green as white due to a
color vision deficiency.

Dual Intensity. Other deficiencies in present-day tail lighting are
the use of the same intensity for daytime brake and turn signaling as is
used at night and the use of chromium and bright trim surrounding and
covering over the tail lights (see Figure 8-19). Even the use of bright red
paint for automobile colors makes an already inadequate daytime brake
light virtually useless. A red brake light surrounded by red paint of an
equal or greater intensity in the daytime cannot have any attraction or
warning value unless one is looking directly at the brake light when it
appears. Tail and brake lights that brighten as the daylight increases are

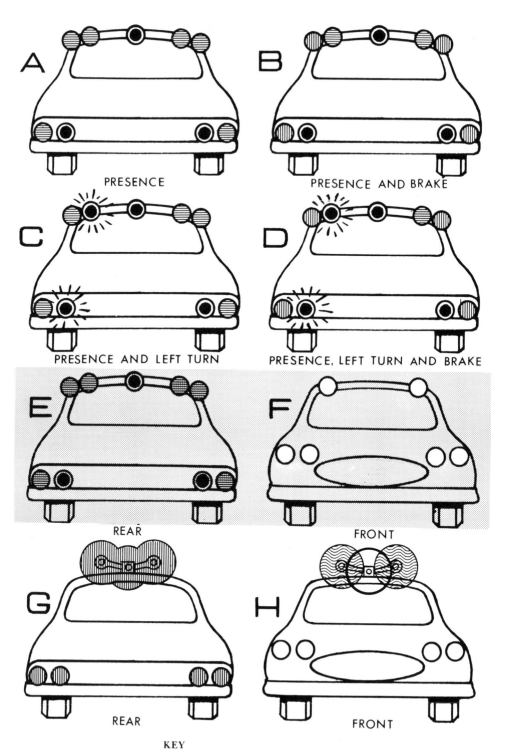

A PRESENCE

B PRESENCE AND BRAKE

C PRESENCE AND LEFT TURN

D PRESENCE, LEFT TURN AND BRAKE

E REAR

F FRONT

G REAR

H FRONT

KEY
Unlit lights—horizontal stripes
Red lights—vertical stripes
Green lights—solid black
Amber lights—wavy line

the answer and are well within automotive technological capabilities. Certainly there can be no objection to leaving off expensive bright trim near the lamps to help their visibility.

FLASH RATE. Special attention must be directed toward signal lights that now flash at pleasant frequencies rather than efficient frequencies. At present, flash rates of 120 per minute or less are the Society of Automotive Engineers' recommendations. Old flashers and bulbs often combine to give flash rates of 10 to 15 per minute. Such a slow rate gives the light an on and an off phase of about 2.5 seconds each. Since a visual fixation takes only 0.20 to 0.25 second, a person could look at a light four or five times, always catch it in the dark or light phase, and thus not be sure it was flashing. Preliminary study indicates that a light that flashes with a short off phase and a relatively long on phase, flashing four to eight times per second, gives a turn signal that is a great deal more effective than the current system.

DIRT. Finally, a major defect in modern automobile rear-end lighting is dirt. Styling dictates changes in lamp housing details, but changes to reduce dirt pickup and moisture penetration are not made because the production run of a particular style is too short. The collection of dust and road mud is a function of position and air flow past the light (see Figure 8-20). Attention to air flow patterns should be a part of lighting design as well as a factor in wind resistance and effective lateral body area distribution. Until such is the case, the motorist and the trucker must make a lamp cleaning tour around his vehicle at each stop.

Water penetration is so severe that tail lights have been observed to be half or more full of water! Even slight water and dust penetration spoils the efficiency of the retroreflector prism faces on the inside of the plastic lens. Paint and plastic materials deposited on the inside of the plastic lens from the heat of the lamp further destroy the retroreflector ef-

Figure 8-18. Various recommended tail and front lighting combinations. In A, triangular green light arrangement denotes the rear end and gives location clues as well as increased visibility in freeway traffic. B shows the more rectangular shape provided by the four red brake lights. In C, flashing of outside presence (green) light and the repeater light at the roof line would give highly visible indication of intent to turn. D shows the degree of isolation of brake, turn, and presence lights. E and F show the impossibility of confusing the proposed rear lighting from the front lighting recommended in Figure 8-15, a consideration dictated by color-blind individuals. G and H show a commercially available roof-mounted system, Safe Lite (Safe Lite, 1969), that approximates the system recommended in A-E. There are three red lights at the roof line. The center is a red presence light that comes on with the ignition. The outside red lights come on for brake operation and flash unilaterally for turn, repeating the normal turn signal. From the front view (H), the center white light is a presence light that comes on with the ignition switch. The two lateral amber lights come on when brakes are applied and flash unilaterally, repeating the turn signal. (A 69-percent reduction in reportable accidents was found among eighty-seven drivers who installed this light system for driving in and around Des Moines, Iowa [Brown, 1969]).

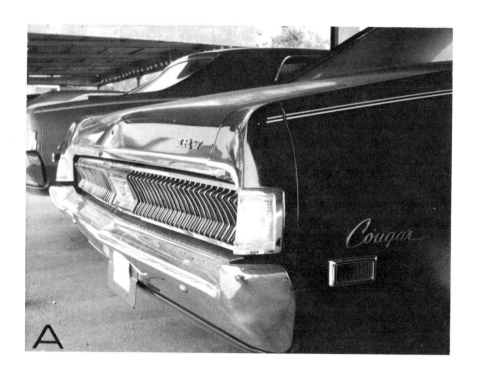

A

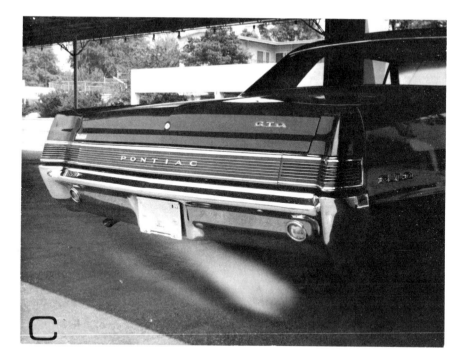

C

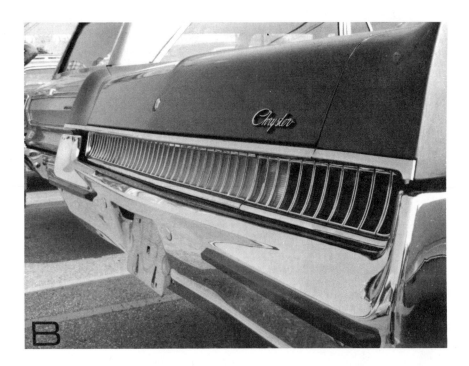

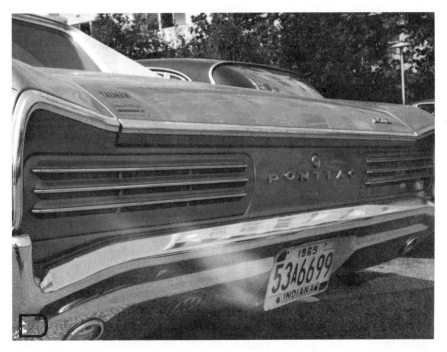

Figure 8-19. Red tail-lighting lenses covered over and camouflaged with chromium and body metal. Daytime signaling can be obliterated by reflections from the bumper or covering grillwork. D shows that body color is displayed right over the tail lamps. When the body paint is bright red, the signal value of the brake or turn lights can go almost to zero in bright sunshine.

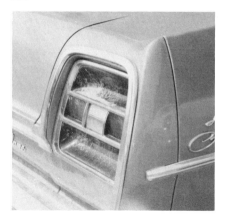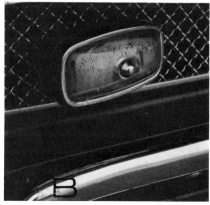

Figure 8-20. Dust and water attenuation of signal lights. A shows complication of design in which more dust collects on the tail light lens than on any other part of the body. B shows moisture penetration into a front turn signal. The author has repeatedly observed water sloshing about in tail light housings. Aerodynamic considerations during design, combined with sealed-beam-type brake, turn, and presence lights, would solve both problems.

ficiency. Moisture damage to painted or aluminized reflective surfaces and moisture-caused corrosion on lamp base contacts and rusted ground connections are of importance in reducing lamp light output. *Sealed unit* tail, brake, and turn lamps, like sealed-beam head lamps, are needed to correct many of these moisture and dirt problems. Such units will also standardize the light output and the shape and the size of the lamp, a much-needed improvement.

VEHICLE VISIBILITY

After over fifty years of manufacturing automobiles in all conceivable colors, the automobile manufacturers still produce car colors in terms of what it is believed will sell, not what is safe. The statistics on accidents surely have been available to the big companies, statistics revealing that light-colored automobiles have fewer accidents than dark. Studies have shown that up to ten times as many accidents happen to black cars as to white. Other data indicate white cars are up to forty times more visible than black (see Figure 8-21). Still other data indicate that greater visibility means fewer and less severe accidents. Red and black have the lowest visibility of all colors. Cream, yellow, and white are the most visible.

Along with statistics on color, it is known that the small, powerful sports car has the highest accident rate and greatest death rate compared to full-sized automobiles. The higher death rate is no surprise because of the small amount of protective metal surrounding the driver. In fact, one

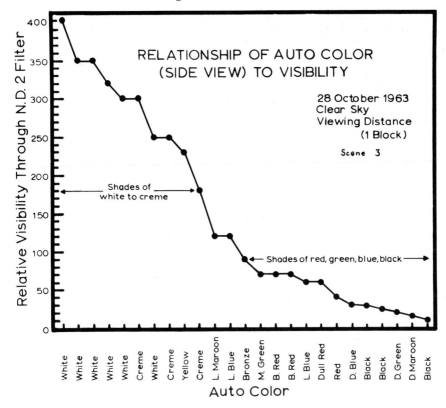

Figure 8-21. Actual field measurements with a Luckiesh-Moss visibility meter of automobile color visibility. Automobiles were observed from a position in front about 45 degrees off the line of travel, much as would be the case in a developing intersection collision. Without question the shades of red, green, blue, and black were more camouflaged than the shades of yellow, cream, and white.

especially hazardous machine is fashioned out of fiberglass, which does not absorb collision energy by crumpling, as sheet metal does. The higher accident rate could be due to speed alone, but indications are that speed is only an indirect factor. The most probable causes of more sports car accidents are the use of dark colors, including the popular red sports car color, and the generally small size (see Figure 8-22). We recognize an object's nearness in part by its size, and we recognize its approach speed almost entirely by the rate of increase in size. Therefore, a small vehicle is judged to be farther away and its approach speed is judged to be slower than it really is. The driver of a sports car cannot rely upon the help of those other drivers who reduce the overall number of accidents by compensating for the mistakes of others. The sports car driver, with his low vantage position, excessive speed potential, low visibility, and a

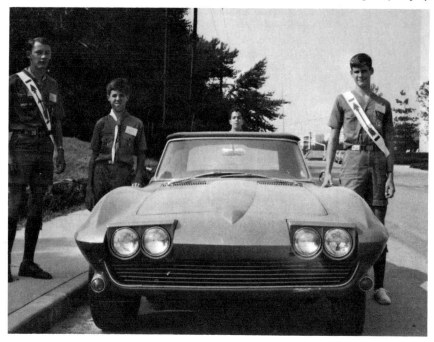

Figure 8-22. An illustration of the low eye height designed into both american and foreign sports cars. Keep in mind that most drivers would be able to look out beneath the rear-view mirror. Note also that there is no visibility through the car due to an aged plastic rear window.

reduction of the amount of Good Samaritan protection from other drivers, must rely almost entirely upon his own skills to avoid accidents. Obviously, from the accident statistics and insurance rates, his own skills alone are not always enough.

It is hoped that the automobile manufacturers will find it expedient to protect the motoring public from the misfit sports car by equipping sports cars with powerful running lights, by painting them with light colors for daytime safety, and by installing full-sized head, tail, and brake lights at normal locations for nighttime use. The sports car driver should be given a higher seating position and an effective, safe periscope which raises his eye level still more. The greater the horsepower, the more hazardous becomes the visual handicaps that are currently built into many sports cars; hence meticulous attention to good visual engineering is imperative.

Since sports car accidents are only a small part of all accidents (because of their small number), it is hoped that manufacturers will soon adopt light colors and daytime running lights for all production vehicles, including trucks, buses, and passenger cars.

Chapter 9: Visual Hazards on Streets and Highways

NIGHTTIME HAZARDS

INADEQUATE ILLUMINATION AND BLACKTOP PAVEMENTS

THE HUMAN EYE is capable of an extreme range of adaptation to changes in the ambient light level. However, such flexibility does not tell the whole story. A major part of this adaptability comes from the ability to change the "grain" of the retina; that is, to group photoreceptors and bipolar, ganglion, and other cells into larger functional units as the light level falls, and into smaller units as the light level rises. The result is a dependency of visual acuity upon light level. See Figure 9-1.

Other important visual functions such as color vision, speed of perception reaction time, binocular fusion, and stereopsis are adversely affected by the increasing retinal grain at lower luminance levels. The contrast sensitivity also is degraded and is of importance in detecting objects as distinct from their background. The greater the contrast sensitivity, the easier it is to detect an object. Figure 9-2 shows the minimum contrast of an object which will make it perceptible at each luminance level. Contrast is defined by the equation

$$C = \frac{B_1 - B_2}{B_1}$$

where C is the contrast, B_1 is the background luminance, and B_2 is the test object luminance. *Contrast sensitivity* is the reciprocal of *contrast*.

Increasing illumination increases the sensitivity to contrast and makes object detection easier. Conversely, Figure 9-2 shows that at nighttime roadway luminance levels of 1 foot-lambert or less an object must be considerably brighter or darker than its background to be seen. Thus objects are more difficult to resolve, as in reading road signs, and the detection of the mere presence of an object such as a pedestrian becomes more difficult. Also—the times for detection, recognition, and response are all increased.

Since the amount of light present is the distinguishing difference be-

141

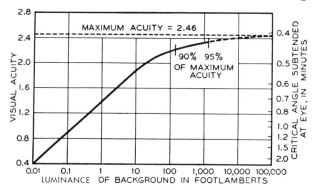

Figure 9-1.   The effect of illumination on visual acuity. A high-contrast black Landolt ring was displayed on a variable luminance background and was observed with normal pupils and binocular vision. (From *IES Lighting Handbook*, 4th ed., Fig. 2-14, p. 2-8.) (Note: The dotted extension of the curve is somewhat misleading as the acuity does not rise past about 900 fL, and 20,000 fL is reported to be intolerable to the eye.)

tween night and day, the problems of night driving would be reduced if more light were available. It has been shown that visibility even in the daytime is improved by adding lights to vehicles (Allen, May 1964, March 1965; Port of New York Authority, 1968). That more light at night is beneficial, using the same system of automobile and highway headlighting as we now have, is predicted from the behavior of the human eye with changing light levels (see Figures 9-1 and 9-2). This has been verified by a number of studies (Roper and Meese, 1964; Christie, 1968) involving accident experience vs. highway lighting and field testing of vehicles with increased headlight output.

Because of the need for more light at night, the blacktop (asphalt) highway, due to its low reflectance, is an uninspired design. The amount of light returned from headlight beams depends upon the composition and aging of the blacktop surface and may vary from virtually zero when the pavement is new or wet to nearly the same as Portland concrete when the blacktop mixture includes a large proportion of light-colored stone and the asphaltic cement has been worn away. Much of seeing at night is by silhouette or backlighting; that is, a dark object is seen against a light background. Portland cement thus gives good visibility because it provides a light background for objects. Pedestrians usually wear dark clothing and are best seen in silhouette; hence blacktopped roadways impair the seeing of pedestrians by drivers. Any light-colored object will stand out better on black, but unfortunately not many roadway hazards are light in color, and few are as important as the pedestrian.

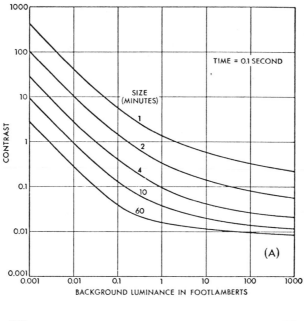

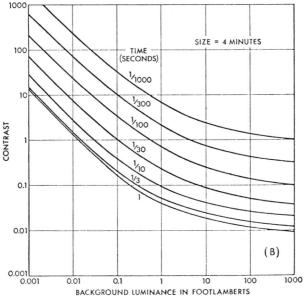

Figure 9-2. The relationship between size, contrast, background luminance, and exposure duration for threshold seeing. Contrast is $\Delta L/L$ where L is the luminance of the background and ΔL is the difference between the luminance of the target and the background. Contrasts above 100 are possible when the test object is brighter than the background. (From *IES Lighting Handbook*, 4th ed., Fig. 2-16, p. 2-8.)

Blacktopped highways also pose a serious physiological threat to night drivers by reducing the total amount of light returned to the eye. A person's alertness depends upon the amount of stimulation he receives. When alone on a highway at night, the lowered light level at his eyes, especially from newly blacktopped roads, makes him less alert and more prone to fall asleep than would be the case with a clean Portland cement highway or a worn, light-colored-aggregate asphaltic highway.

On the positive side for blacktopped pavements, many states use reflectorized paint in the center and along the edges of the pavement. The bright edge of the pavement then stands out in sharp contrast to the dark surface. These reflectorized lines are a very great assistance to night driving because they make the task of staying on the roadway in the proper lane easily possible in the face of the greatest amounts of glare. In addition, continuous edge marking will help reveal a pedestrian on the pavement near the right edge of the roadway at comfortably safe distances by silhouette lighting.

With the onset of rain the advantage of blacktop disappears in supplying contrast to edge and center reflectorized paint lines. Wet blacktop pavement becomes even blacker, and the currently used reflectorized paint loses most of its unique properties. The film of water prevents headlight rays, which approach at grazing incidence, from penetrating to the detail of the roadway; furthermore it defocuses the beads used in the reflectorized paint. Hence at the time when headlights put out less useful light, due to dirt and raindrop scatter, and cause more glare to oncoming motorists because of reflections from the pavement and from dirt and raindrop scatter, and when the light scattered from dirt, condensation, and rain water droplets on the windshield is at a maximum, the blacktop pavement itself and its markings are significantly less visible. On the other hand, the glossy surface reflectance when pavements are wet effectively extends the headlight range, and objects placed in the roadway may be illuminated at greater than normally expected distances and thus may be as visible as when the pavement, windshield, and headlights are dry.

The motorist's ability to localize his own vehicle properly in his own lane is seriously impaired because of loss of edge detail when the blacktop pavement is wet and because of the obscuring power of the rain droplets in the atmosphere. The amount of obscuration due to rain is not dependent on the size of the rain drops but on the number of drops falling on a unit of area in one second (Middleton, 1958). Stated in another way, obscuration depends upon the number of drops per unit volume of air at any given instant. The combination effect on vision of drop obscuration in the atmosphere, water splatter pattern on the windshield, and back scatter of light from the headlights by water drops in the air near the driver's line of sight has never been quantified to the author's knowledge. However, one knows from experience that the result is a seeing condition that is unusually poor and hazardous.

IMPROPER USE OF REFLECTORS

The retroreflector, composed of internally reflecting prisms called *cube corners,* is one of the most useful protective devices ever invented. Placed on automobiles, bicycles, trucks, trains, and pedestrians, the result is a three- to tenfold increase in the distance at which the objects can be detected. However, a retroreflector as popularly used becomes just a spot of light in a field of blackness until the motorist is near enough to have his headlights reveal the nature of the object supporting the reflector. To aid in quick identification, reflectors placed on the rear of vehicles are red (except for reflectorized license plates) and those near the front currently and incorrectly are amber. To identify the type of vehicle or even where it is requires the motorist to approach close enough for headlighting to reveal the details. The goal of marking a vehicle by reflectors is to provide a passive system at night that always reveals its presence and location.

Unfortunately, things do not work so well in practice because of a general lack of understanding of retroreflectors and how to use them. For example, nonhazardous driveways along a roadway are often marked with red reflectors, while bridge abutments within inches of high-speed traffic, even on new interstate highways, are not reflectorized. A person may wish to identify his own driveway and he should be permitted to do so, but not with red, which is supposed to mean danger.

Another example is the highway delineators which are retroreflectors on top of four-foot steel posts placed parallel to the edge of the roadway. The retroreflector color is normally white, with amber being used to mark exit ramps on divided highways, thus duplicating the reflector color on the front of an automobile or truck. Since the eye level of the driver of a modern automobile rarely exceeds 48 inches, most motorists must look up to see these reflectors. If the road curves, they can see the curve only by the apparent changes in reflector spacing and by the fact that the reflectors that are the farthest away are the least bright. The normally powerful perspective cues, such as the curve of the edge of the road and the lower object being nearer, are completely missing or are reversed if the reflectors are above the driver's eye level. At 48 inches in height the reflectors are in a less intense portion of the headlight beam pattern and hence cannot reflect much light. The ideal location for such reflectors is at the edge and attached to the surface of the pavement. If they must be moved back into the grass they should be placed within 12 inches of the ground. Perhaps the four-foot post is needed to prevent a mower from striking it, but the reflectors should be near the bottom. The presence of these delineator posts is an unnecessary obstruction. They are often struck, generally provide no useful information, and the reflectors divert the eyes from the road and are often deceptive. To ensure their low visibility, the posts themselves are usually painted a pretty, camouflaging green!

Reflectors placed on trucks and on slow-moving vehicles are usually too high for accurate localization by perspective clues. In fact, on trucks the narrow spacing of lights and reflectors often encountered, plus the dirt and the high placement, may deceive even the sophisticated motorist into believing that a slower-moving truck is far away when in reality a collision may be imminent. Many rear-end accident drivers show little or no effort to brake prior to collision, and in many instances the motorist has actually left the highway, following the lights of a parked vehicle to collide with it.

There are two classes of retroreflectors used on automotive equipment. Class A retroreflectors are defined by their light output distribution and intensity, which are given in the following table:

TABLE 9-1
MINIMUM CANDLEPOWER PER INCIDENT FOOT-CANDLE
FOR CLASS A RED REFLEX REFLECTOR

Observation	Entrance Angles, Degrees				
Angle, Degrees	0	10 Up	10 Down	20 Left	20 Right
0.2	4.5	3.0	3.0	1.5	1.5
1.5	0.07	0.05	0.05	0.03	0.03

The *incidence angle* is the angle formed by the incident light beam with the normal to the surface of the reflective device, e.g., a sign or license plate; or from the optic axis, e.g., a tail light lens with integral retroreflector.

The *observation* (*divergence*) *angle* is the angle formed by the observer's line of sight and the illuminating beam where these two lines intersect at the reflector.

A Class B retroreflector must meet the requirements shown in the following table:

TABLE 9-2
MINIMUM CANDLEPOWER PER INCIDENT FOOT-CANDLE
FOR CLASS B RED REFLEX REFLECTOR

Observation	Entrance Angles, Degrees				
Angle, Degrees	0	10 Up	10 Down	20 Left	20 Right
0.2	0.50	0.40	0.40	0.20	0.20
1.5	0.01	0.01	0.01	0.01	0.01

The usual size for the Class A and B reflectors is 4 inches in diameter. Thus, the candlepower per square foot of reflector surface is quite high (12.6 times greater than the values given for the 4-inch size). Even though the Class A reflector, especially, has a very high light-returning ability, it does this only along the axis or normal to the surface. At 20 degrees off axis the light returned is down to one third. Hence for wide-angle usage as on the sides of automobiles the Class A reflector must be especially redesigned. Reflective sheeting, on the other hand, is composed of imbedded spheres instead of internally reflecting prisms and has as its great virtue a high efficiency at a large acceptance or entrance angle.

Table 9-3 permits comparisons of reflective sheeting of various colors and efficiencies with cube-corner Class A reflectors.

In Table 9-3 candle power per foot-candle per square foot is a measure of the efficiency of the reflector under certain standard conditions such as a divergence angle of 0.5 degree with an incidence angle of -4 degrees or $+30$ degrees, as used in retroreflective license plate testing. The following formula gives the essential relationships:

$$CP_R = \frac{I_R \cdot d^2}{I_E \cdot A}$$

CP_R is the candle power of the reflector, I_R is the illumination falling on the plane of the reflector in foot-candles, d is the distance between the source of illumination and the reflector, I_E is the illumination falling on the eye or the photodetector in foot-candles returned from the reflector, and A is the area of the reflector in square feet.

The Federal Motor Vehicle Safety Standards (U.S. Department of Transportation, 1968) calls for Class A retroreflectors for rear application and Class A retroreflectors or reflective sheeting for side markers. The higher light output at high incidence angles makes the reflective sheeting well suited for side marker use, since a vehicle is vulnerable from all angles. Unless the cube-corner-type (Class A and B) reflectors are especially constructed, they cannot give the coverage angles needed. Special side marker cube-corner-type reflectors have been developed and are adequate for the wide-angle coverage needed. They thus exceed the Society of Automotive Engineers' Class A requirements for incidence angle in the horizontal meridian and begin to equal the performance of reflective sheeting in this respect. It appears from the table that reflective sheeting is both comparable in performance to cube-corner reflectors and has definite advantages at high-incidence angles.

TABLE 9-3

COMPARATIVE BRIGHTNESS OF 3M SCOTCHLITE BRAND SHEETING AND CUBE-CORNER REFLECTORS

(candle power per foot-candle per square foot)

Incidence Angle Degree	Divergence Angle Degree	3070 (3M) White	3170 (3M) White	3270 (3M) Silver	3870 (3M) Silver	3M Signal Del. Silver	SAE Class A Cube Corner (White)	3171 (3M) Yellow	3271 (3M) Yellow	3274 (3M) Orange	3870 Type Amber (3M)	3M Signal Del.-Amber	SAE Class B Cube Corner (Amber)	3272 (3M) Red	3870 Type Red (3M)	3M Signal Red	SAE Class A Cube Corner (Red)
−4	0.2	30	45	60	155	187	224	25	30	16	60	112	140	12.5	30	56	56
+10	0.2			55	100	180	144		25	15		108	90	11.5		54	36
+15	0.2			50	50	173	72		25	13.5	42	104	45	10.5	21	52	18
+20	0.2	7.0	7.5	40	25	144		5.5	20	11		86		8.5		43	
+30	0.2			25	10	72			15	7	17	43		5.5	8.5	21	
+40	0.2			12.5					6.0	2.8	6			1.9	3.0		
+45	0.2			5.0					4.0	2.5				1.5			
+50	0.2			3.5					2.5	1.2				0.9			
−4	0.5	18	23	25	65	72		12.5	15	8	20	43		6.5	10	21	
+10	0.5			25	50	72			14	7.5		43		6.0		21	
+15	0.5			25	25	65			12	6.5	17	39		5.5	8.5	19	
+20	0.5	4.5	5.0	20	15	50		3.0	10	5.5		30		4.5		15	
+30	0.5			15	5.0	29			8	3.5	10	17		3.0	5.0	8.5	
+40	0.5			7.5					4	2.0	2.5			1.2	1.2		
+45	0.5			3.5					2.8	1.2				1.0			
+50	0.5			3.0					1.5	0.5				0.4			
−4	1.5	2.5	3.0	4.0	8		3.4	2.0	2.5	1.2			2.1	1.0			.84
+10	1.5			3.5			2.4		2.5	1.1			1.5	0.9			.60
+15	1.5			3.0			1.4		2.5	1.0			0.9	0.8			.36
+20	1.5	1.5	1.5	2.5	2.0			0.8	2.3	0.8				0.7			
+30	1.5			2.0					1.8	0.5				0.5			
+40	1.5			1.6					0.9	0.4				0.4			
+45	1.5			1.1					0.8	0.2				0.1			
+50	1.5			1.1					0.5	0.1				0.1			

Highway reflectorized paint is a different problem, as will be seen in Figure 9-3. This figure details the role played by the left and right head-lights in the typical automobile at the upper limit of the low-beam head lamps. Since the 300 feet is not to scale with the height and spacing of the lamps, the angles are not true; however, they do indicate the grazing nature of the illuminating and viewing rays. Such tiny angles make the measurement especially difficult. Figure 9-4 shows the optics of a portable pavement-marking photometer built by the 3M Company. Note the folded light path needed to make the optical path long enough to permit reasonable aperture spacings to provide the 0.33-degree and 0.78-degree angles between the incident and view rays.

Figure 9-5 gives the aging characteristics of three different beaded paint stripes exposed to highway traffic as measured by the 3M instrument and the Hunter Night Visibility Meter, a fairly widely used instrument. Paint reflectance varies as beads wear away and new beads are exposed, which is not necessarily a linear effect.

A different device has been employed by the author to make paint stripe measurements. It uses the highly versatile Pritchard Spectrophotometer (Photo Research Corporation) as a photodetector and an automobile bulb as a light source. The optics are similar to those in a retinoscope. They are cheap, rugged, and self-aligning.

PEDESTRIANS—A DOUBLE HAZARD AND A DOUBLE RIGHT

A pedestrian has the right to be protected from careless motorists. Similarly, a motorist has a right to be protected from careless pedestrians.

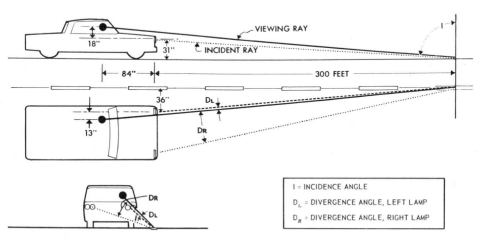

Figure 9-3. Relationship between driver, head lamps, and pavement marking. Geometry involved in reflectivity from center-line point at 300 feet distance, using representative dimensions for a dual head lamp vehicle. (From Harrington et al., 1962.)

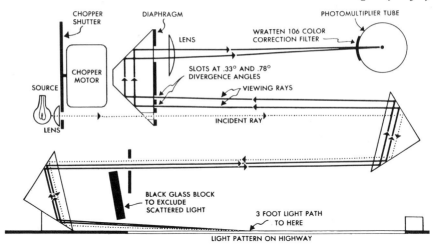

Figure 9-4. Principal components of new pavement-marking photometer optical system. (From Harrington et al., 1962.)

That headlights at night do provide the pedestrian with warning of an approaching automobile as well as helping the motorist is indicated by the report of a 14.1-percent drop in pedestrian-vehicle accidents after the change-over was made to low-beam headlights instead of parking lights within the New York City limits on February 4, 1952.

Unfortunately, the motorist usually has no warning of the presence of a pedestrian because of the normal low reflectivity of clothing. An illustration of the difficulty is the following incident which occurred early in our testing of pedestrian visibility. The experimenters found that cardboard boxes, spray-painted black, were visible at considerable distances because of surface reflections. To evaluate quickly the visibility of cloth, one of the graduate students volunteered to stand in the roadway while a second student approached in an automobile at 20 miles per hour. The plan was to stop as soon as the driver saw the pedestrian's dark clothing. The pedestrian stood in line with the driver's side of the approaching car and waited, anticipating the driver's stop. It finally became necessary to leap out of the way as the car continued down the road at 20 miles per hour. When the driver returned to the pedestrian's location, he asked, "Where were you?" A simple question indeed, but one of great significance. Keep in mind the slow speed, the motorist's sure knowledge that a pedestrian was out there, the absence of glare, and the driver's ready-to-stop attitude.

In the nighttime pedestrian accident reports on record in the Indiana Department of Motor Vehicles for 1966, 87 percent of the drivers

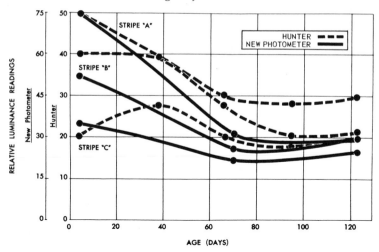

Figure 9-5. Relative luminance readings vs. age of reflectorized highway paint. Comparison of reflectorized transverse test stripes for three representative 1.5 index beaded markings as measured by the Hunter and the New Photometer. (Wisconsin highway department annual performance test stripes.) (From Harrington, et al., 1962.)

whose automobile struck a pedestrian at night claimed difficulty in seeing the pedestrian, while only 11.8 percent made the same claim during the daytime. Furthermore, 23.4 percent of the drivers at night claimed they heard the impact before they saw the pedestrian!

Since the percentage of blood alcohol is higher among dead pedestrians than among the population at risk at the same location as the accident (Haddon et al., 1961; Indiana University, 1964), pedestrians obviously are not always able to avoid an automobile even though headlights do offer a warning. The motorist also deserves some warning sign to help protect the pedestrian and to protect himself. There are signs that announce a curve ahead, road repairs in progress, a dead end, or a stop sign, but the sign that flashes only when a pedestrian is present has not yet been invented.

Table 9-4 gives the reaction distance plus the stopping distance, called critical visibility distance, for an automobile, with safe tires and brakes, traveling on dry pavement and driven by an individual with a reaction time of 0.75 seconds.*

* A recent study (Mortimer, 1968) indicates that the reaction time is about one second in highway experiments. One can confidently expect a nonexperimental driver to have a much longer reaction time.

TABLE 9-4

Miles Per Hour	Critical Visibility Distance (ft.)
20	45
30	72
40	123
50	185
60	261
70	349
80	450

Table 9-5 indicates the percentage of pedestrians, "Ps," who were safely visible at distances greater than the critical visibility distance associated with the given speeds. There was no opposing glare.

Table 9-6 indicates the percentage of pedestrians who were safely visible at distances greater than the critical visibility distance associated with the given speeds. The data are from four observers after the consumption of alcohol (blood alcohol level from 0.06% to 0.10%). There was no opposing glare. This reversal in Tables 9-5 and 9-6 between drunk and sober is probably due to the small sample and to statistical fluctuations.

The pedestrians' cloth reflectances were as follows: black, 9 percent; gray, 16 percent; white, 75 percent; and reflectorized tape 1 inch wide by 12 inches long of 50 candles per square foot per foot-candle of illumination. The "pedestrian" was a tall cardboard box, 1 foot by 1 foot by 4 feet, covered with cloth.

TABLE 9-5

	Miles Per Hour						
	20	30	40	50	60	70	80
Black P	86.4%	68.2%	45.4%	15.9%	0 %	0 %	0 %
Gray P	100	100	47.2	13.9	5.5	5.5	0
White P	100	100	100	100	97.2	91.7	52.7
Reflectorized P	100	100	100	100	100	100	100

TABLE 9-6

	Miles per hour						
	20	30	40	50	60	70	80
Black P	90.8%	63.6%	15.2%	0 %	0 %	0 %	0 %
Gray P	97.2	73.2	14.2	2.7	0	0	0
White P	100	100	94.4	88.9	80.5	61.1	25
Reflectorized P	100	100	100	100	100	100	94.5

In evaluating tables 9-5 and 9-6 one must realize that a 97 percent probability of seeing 100 pedestrians in time still leaves 3 that were not seen in time! Thus the black "P" seems safe up to 20 miles per hour, especially if the driver is sober and no oncoming glare is present. However, Table 9-6 shows that if the driver is under the influence of alcohol (0.06-0.10 percent) but not legally drunk (0.15 percent in many states), he will fail to see in time some pedestrians dressed in white at only 40 miles per hour, which is at the bottom limit of speed of most highway traffic even at night.

Since men traditionally wear dark clothing, and since twice as many men are killed as women, who tend to dress more colorfully, clothing appears to be a factor in accident statistics. However, more men are at risk than women, and such a conclusion is somewhat speculative. Because of the naturally dark nature of male pedestrians' clothes and their demonstrated poor visibility at night, some protective device such as a retroreflector is a necessity to protect the pedestrian and to give the motorist some peace of mind.

Tables 9-5 and 9-6 show the remarkable benefit from a 1-by-12-inch piece of cloth, factory treated with reflective beads. The cloth appears silver gray until a light near the observer's line of sight illuminates it; then it appears brightly glowing. Pedestrian protection also could be provided by using reflectorized buttons, shoe reflectors, or reflectorized dangle tags.

The motorist who has just been demoted to pedestrian status by a flat tire, for example, could obtain increased visibility at night by using a side lamp directed to light the ground around the vehicle. About 1928, L. D. Bridge was issued a patent on a Safety Side Light to assist people entering and leaving an automobile. It provided considerable light for tire repairs, for illuminating the pedestrian, for localization of the vehicle, for entering driveways, and even was of some benefit in fogs. These lights were not adopted for passenger automobiles, though General Motors now has a cornering light that resembles the original Bridge light.

In 1926 Charles A. Sims invented the Sims Side Lamp (see Figure 9-6). His announcement began, "The Sims Side Lamp. At Last! After thousands have sacrificed their lives, after science has dug deep, and industry spent fortunes, a simple idea solves the glaring headlight trouble." His idea was never taken up by the auto industry, either. Decisions about headlighting were made, but they were for the high-low-beam headlight system we have today.

Without knowledge of the work of these early inventors, the author proposed a side light system (Allen, October 1962) to light the way for the oncoming driver. This involved lights in a number of positions, including the top of the car. The most efficient was at bumper height, aimed backward to light the pavement adjacent to the test vehicle. Fig-

ure 9-7 shows lights mounted on the front bumper on each side. The rear
fender behind the rear wheel is probably the optimum place to set the
light into the body work. The light on the right side is of some benefit,
but practical considerations might limit the system only to the lights at
the left rear. Figures 9-8 and 9-9 show the benefits of the system in over-
coming the glare of oncoming automobiles.

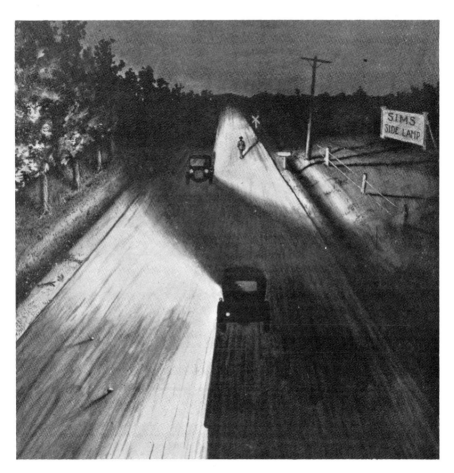

Figure 9-6. Side lamps for aiding oncoming motorist, patented by Charles Sims,
January 10, 1928. Mr. Sims described the intended method of operation as follows: "As
shown above when two cars approach each other the operators switch OFF their front
lights entirely, and automatically switch ON the side lights which illuminates the roadway for each other. Instead of shooting the light AT each other, you reverse it and shoot
it FROM each other. It's done instantly without vibration or flickering, no refocusing of the
eyes to penetrate a different degree of light or darkness. You are still looking after the
light and not into it." (Taken from materials describing the Sims patent, with permission.)

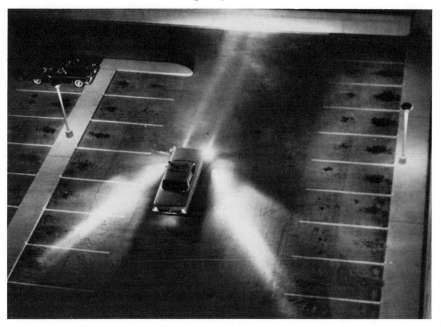

Figure 9-7. Backward-aimed headlights to aid the oncoming driver. A 5½-inch sealed-beam headlight was mounted on the front bumper at each side. These lights were aimed backward as shown. The lower and more nearly straight back they were placed, the better they lighted the pavement for the oncoming driver.

The idea for such a system came from using the light spilled laterally across the road by earlier automobile headlights. Modern headlight design and wrap-around fenders have eliminated this weak but very valuable clue. In fact, the modern shielding of head and tail lights from side view prompted the General Services Administration and later the Department of Transportation to require *both* side marker lights *and* reflectors on all new passenger cars, trucks, and buses by 1970.

Considerable experience was gained using the side light system shown in Figure 9-7. Twenty automobiles were equipped and sent out on a quiet highway in a caravan. Motion pictures were taken of the effects of meeting, passing, and following such vehicles. The results were considered to be highly favorable. The system is recommended as a means of providing glare-free illumination on the streets and highways which increases as traffic increases and does not require the cost and upkeep of extensive stationary highway lighting. This is not a proposal to do away with conventional highway lighting or the very high-mounted lighting advocated by the Texas Transportation Institute, but such lighting can never be everywhere or enough. The side lighting would provide am-

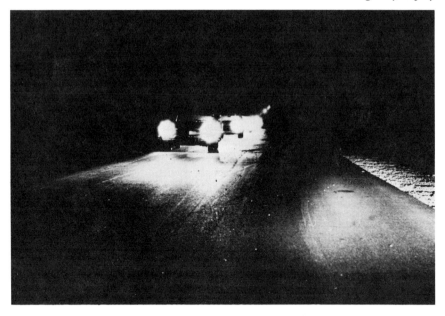

Figure 9-8. Unseen pedestrians stand on the pavement beside four approaching cars on low beams. The camera car's low beams do not reveal the presence of the hazard.

bient light when needed to reveal pedestrians and other road hazards. It would be turned off automatically when no cars were present. The lone motorist operating on high beams is reasonably able to see hazards if speeds are not excessive. As soon as he dropped to low beams because of other automobiles, his side lights would come on to help oncoming motorists; at the same time the aproaching motorists' side lights would come on when they dimmed *their* lights.

Rain and Fog Hazards

Water particles between 2 and 100 microns are found in fog. Figure 9-10 shows that for practical purposes fog is not found with particle sizes less than about 10 microns, and this only in clouds.

Particles below 2 microns produce haze. Water particles do not exist below about 0.2 microns, as seen in figure 9-11.

Fog and cloud particles act to scatter visible light uniformly without regard to wavelength. Even haze does not scatter blue and green much more than red. Rayleigh's theory of light scatter leads to the following equation

$$s = 24\pi^3 \left(\frac{n^2 - 1}{n^2 + 2} \right) \frac{V^2}{\lambda^4}$$

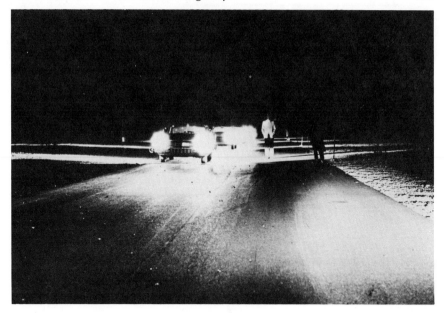

Figure 9-9. Silhouette and direct lighting provided by side lights. The three pedestrians now become visible. Note the increased size of the field of view compared to Figure 9-8. The driver of a side-lighted automobile finds the increase in peripheral field of view a help in maintaining orientation and alertness.

where s is the total scattered light from a unit intensity of illumination of wavelength λ, n is the refractive index, and V is the volume of the particle. Table 9-7 derived from Rayleigh's theory gives the relative amounts of scattering by clean dry air at 1013.2 millibar pressure and 0 degrees Centigrade temperature for each wavelength, λ, in nanometers.

TABLE 9-7

λ	400	500	600	700
Relative scatter	4.358	1.750	0.833	0.466
Loss at 800 meters	3.2%	1.4%	0.67%	0.361%

Rayleigh scatter holds for spherical particles up to 0.1 wavelength. As the particle sizes increase, the scattering function becomes more complex; and for certain particle sizes it is possible even to have more red scatter than blue. However, in general, clean atmospheric transmission favors the longer wavelengths. The table above shows that for automobile travel this is probably of no significance because of the short ranges usually involved, less than 0.50 mile (800 meters).

The smallest cloud particles are encountered in stratus clouds which average 4 microns, with cumulus clouds averaging 5 microns and nimbostratus, 10 microns (Middleton, 1958). These sizes are significantly larger

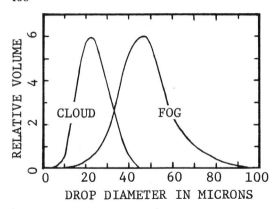

Figure 9-10. Typical drop-size distributions for a costal fog and for a cloud (mountain fog). The curves are plotted to show how the liquid water is distributed (by volume) among the various drop sizes. (After Houghton [1939], from Middleton [1958], Figure 3-18.)

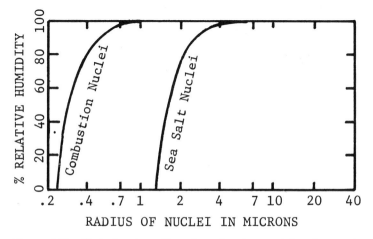

Figure 9-11. Variation in radius of combustion nuclei and sea salt nuclei with relative humidity. (After Wright [1939], from Middleton [1958], Figure 3-1.)

than the .55-micron wavelength of visible light; hence selective absorption of various wavelengths is practically nonexistent. Certainly, the average ground fog with particle sizes from 15 to 100 microns will act impartially upon all visible wavelengths. Thus, automobile fog light color has no scientific basis, and the superior performance claimed for fog lights must result from secondary factors such as the narrow beam spread and remote location of the beam from the line of sight. Similarly, arguments as to the benefits or disadvantages of one color over another in penetrating fog or rain have no substance for automobile signal systems. A proper signal system can be chosen only after evaluating the physiological, psychological, and systems aspects of the driving problem.

Daytime fog is dangerous for driving because it scatters, or attenuates, the useful light coming from the object and substitutes random light from elsewhere. This reduces the contrast of the object without changing the sharpness of its borders. Increasing distance increases the attenuation of the useful light and increases the veiling light added. The attenuation function is that of any filter; that is, a percentage is lost per unit of distance the light travels. The veiling effect, however, makes the daytime seeing evaluation somewhat more complex, while the nighttime situation involving headlights is even more complex. Without nearby headlights, an automobile's headlights or tail lights can be seen at a considerable distance in fog, because, no matter how dense the fog, theoretically some light will get through to the observer. If the intervening fog is illuminated by one's own headlights, the amount of light coming through the fog from the oncoming automobile must exceed the just noticeable brightness difference at the level of illumination caused by one's own lights. Of course, as fog density goes up, the greater is the nearby fog illumination from one's own lights and the smaller is the amount of light penetrating through the fog from the oncoming car.

The classification of fog is difficult, but Table 9-8 provides an operational definition of the several subjective terms that are often used. The daylight visual range is for the detection of dark objects about the size of an automobile as seen against a light background. The atmospheric transmission is given for each type of fog for various distances and would be useful in calculating the range at which a light could be seen through fog, assuming that the minimum contrast for detection between the light and its background needs to be 4 percent or more.

TABLE 9-8
ATMOSPHERIC TRANSMISSION *

Code No.	Weather	Maximum Daylight Visual Range (ft.)	Maximum Transmission at Ranges Indicated (In %)					
			3280	1640	820	410	205	102
0	Dense fog	164				1×10^{-6}	0.1	3
1	Thick fog	658	32×10^{-8}	.005	.71	8.4	29	54
2	Moderate fog	1640	.004	0.63	7.9	28	53	72
3	Light fog	3280	2	14	37.5	61	78	88
4	Thin fog	6560	14	37.5	61	78	88	94
5	Haze	26,240	37	61	78	88	94	96
6	Light Haze	32,800	68	82	91	95	98	
7	Clear	65,600	82	91	95	98		
8	Very clear	164,000	93	96	98			
9	Extra clear	164,000+	93+					

* Data adapted from IES Handbook, 2nd. ed., 1952, pp. 9–44, Illuminating Engineering Society, 1860 Broadway, New York.

The visibility of roadway details falls off more quickly than is the case for light sources. The following analogy will illustrate the principles involved. If one looks through a handkerchief held very near to his eyes he will be able to see large objects, but will have lost the ability to see detail. The white cloth transmits some light from the objects, but it also is itself an object, brightly illuminated by the ambient light. Now consider that the room is dark and that the objects you are trying to see are illuminated only by the light that has penetrated the handkerchief from a flashlight you hold in your hand. The handkerchief is equivalent to an impenetrable "Fog" and you must change it to something like a nylon stocking of loose mesh to be able to see through to the objects. If you hold the flashlight beyond the handkerchief so it illuminates the objects directly, without illuminating the cloth, visibility is improved.

Thus, a fog light should illuminate no fog between the driver's eye and the object viewed. However, in practice, secondary scattering from fog particle to fog particle and limitations as to where lights can be placed on the car, both limit the performance of a fog light. To achieve the best possible vision in fog, the fog lamp should be low and to the extreme right corner of the vehicle away from the driver. The lamp should produce a concentrated beam with no upward scatter above the horizontal; or, in effect, it should be in a tube about two feet long to eliminate all spill light that could illuminate the fog particles in front of the driver's eyes.

RAILROAD CROSSINGS

Railroad crossings are a significant hazard. The Department of Transportation (DOT, 1968) reports as follows:

Of the 3,932 crossing accidents of all kinds in 1967, 3,733 involved collisions between railroad movements and motor vehicles and resulted in 1,520 deaths and 3,726 injuries. In 2,456 collisions, 65.79 percent, trains struck motor vehicles, resulting in 1,158, or 76.18 percent, of the deaths and in 2,218, or 59.53 percent, of the injuries. In the other 1,277 collisions, 34.21 percent, motor vehicles struck the sides of train movements, resulting in 362, or 23.82 percent, of the deaths and in 1,508, or 40.47 percent, of the injuries.

Of the 3,733 collisions, 1,617, or 43.32 percent, occurred at crossings which were especially protected by one of the following: lowered gates, trainman, watchman, audible and visual signals, audible signals, or visible signals. The other 2,116, or 56.68 percent, occurred at crossings protected by signals or signs that did not indicate the approach of trains.

The latest available statistics show a total of 214,417 rail-highway crossings at grade. Of these crossings, 44,432 or 20.72 percent, were specially protected; 169,985, or 79.28 percent, were not specially protected.

Of the 3,733 crossing collisions, 2,273, or 60.89 percent, occurred in daylight, and 1,460, or 39.11 percent, took place at night. There were 2,564 collisions, or 68.68 percent, in clear weather, and 1,169, or 31.32 percent, under cloudy or inclement weather conditions.

Of the 3,733 collisions between trains and motor vehicles, automobiles were involved in 2,906, or 77.85 percent; busses in 11, or 0.29 percent; motortrucks in 780, or 20.89 percent, and motorcycles in 36, or 0.96 percent.

Very little modern technology has crept into railroading if the signals at 79.28 percent of the intersections are any criterion. At most crossings the only signal present is the typical railroad cross buck. Often only one is present and in design, color, and size of lettering is just as it was years ago. Nevertheless about $190 million per year was spent on railway crossings from 1963 to 1967 (Insurance Institute for Highway Safety 1970).

In the past the railroads have lost few lawsuits and have been slow to make improvements. This is partly because accidents at a particular crossing are infrequent, and partly because it is difficult to convince a jury that a train can be unnecessarily difficult to see and hear. Of course, failure to provide locomotives and rolling stock with maximum visibility paints, reflectors, and lights, as well as failure to keep signs and signals in top condition, can be considered to be contributory negligence in some accidents. Because families and friends of motorists who have died in train accidents have not been able to organize effectively to express their righteous indignation loudly, we continue to live with the hazard.

The problem is manifold. (1) Since we tend to ignore the passive signs at the 79.28 percent of the crossings that do not signal the approach of a train, the active signals at other crossings tend to be ignored as well. (2) On the average the accident probability at a crossing is one every ten years (Schoppert et al., 1968), or so infrequently that it does not seem to be a problem to the local citizens. (3) A fast train on a collision course with an automobile must be looked for at angles ranging from 45 to 90 degrees from straight ahead or, for the most part, must be looked for through the side windows. (4) Trains provide their bulk above the line of sight, so that for a slow or stopped train it is often possible to view a seemingly unobstructed roadway beneath a railroad car, especially at night. (5) Trains are usually not painted in light colors, are not reflectorized, are not lighted, and are not clean. (6) The active as well as the passive railroad crossing signals are archaic and hence not visually designed to use all the clues of spatial localization, maximum visibility, and signal information free of ambiguity.

TRUCKS

Trucks on the streets and highways represent a special hazard to passenger automobile drivers because of their poor visibility. This is another instance of virtual protection or immunity being extended to trucks because of their economic importance and legislative lobbying ability. No lobby of the relatives of the dead is present in the legislative halls to counter truck lobbies. Part of their immunity comes from law. It is a fact that the vehicle striking the rear of another vehicle is held to be at fault automatically unless partially relieved of that fault by contributory negligence on the part of the struck vehicle. So long as the inadequate Interstate Commerce Commission requirements for lights and reflectors on trucks are adhered to, the stopped or slow-moving truck is not held to be contributory, and hence there is little incentive to improve the visibility of trucks. Such protection also leads to inadequate under-run protection, which leads to a high fatality rate for car-truck collisions. Since there are fewer survivors of collisions with the rear or side of a truck compared to other types of collisions, because the passenger vehicle runs under the frame of the truck and shears off the top, the insurance or court proceedings are simpler and the amount of damages claimed are usually less.

Truckers operate their vehicles under the rules of the Interstate Commerce Commission, which seems to work closely with industry to set so-called "realistic" standards, including those for vehicle lighting. That these standards might pose a hazard to passenger vehicles is difficult to prove in a court of law trying to assess who is to blame in a particular accident. Judges and juries are not naturally aware of highway and vehicle design deficiencies and are likely to assume that meeting federal regulations provides the best that there is. Though federal regulations are intended to represent the minimum, they often end up being the maximum in practice.

Federal lighting requirements for 1969 for trucks and trailers of 80 inches or wider are shown in Tables 9-10 and 9-11 (U.S. Department of Transportation, 1968). These standards offer some improvements over standards in effect prior to 1969. For example, two tail lights and turn signals are now required on truck tractors instead of the previous one and none respectively. However, significant inconsistencies persist, such as the amber brake, turn, and hazard warning signals permitted on the rear along with amber park, turn, and hazard warning signals on the front. Retention of other hazardous specifications indicate that more revisions are needed. Such hazardous specifications include permitting headlights to be as high as 54 inches, when the average eye height of an automobile driver is below 48 inches; permission to place tail lights and stop lights as high as 72 inches above the road; permission to place reflex reflectors as high as 60 inches when automobile head lamps are about 28 inches high and aimed downward; permission to place side marker lamps and turn signal lamps anywhere above 15 inches; and the continued use of identification and clearance lights whose respective purposes have little if anything to contribute to safe operation of the trucking equipment in traffic.

The nature of the remaining hazards becomes clear if one encounters a truck-trailer crossing an intersection. The lights at the top are of no value in locating the truck, for they might seem to be, for example, on a television antenna tower miles away. The reflectors on the sides are usually dirty and are above the beams of the standard automobile headlight and most truck headlights as well, because of aiming practices. The side marker lamps have no specified height above 15 inches and most usually are mounted high; hence they are of little utility in localizing the vehicle. Most truck trailers have a high bed permitting unobstructed vision beneath it, especially for those seated in an automobile. Upon seeing the roadway unobstructed, and with the weak ambiguous side lights mounted high overhead, the motorist may be lured into a side collision which will have a high probability of being fatal to him.

From the rear view the hazard is similar. Closely spaced tail lights, as sometimes used, covered with dirt and mounted high, appear to be significantly farther away than they actually are and tend to lure the unwary motorist in too close. If the speed difference is great enough, a collision will result. With his lights on and reflectors in place, the trucker is not legally negligent, but the motorist who died is, even though he couldn't see the truck or misjudged its location and speed. Keeping one's vehicle under control as required by law is one thing, and having a fighting chance to know of the hazard one faces from the low visibility and deceptiveness of modern trucks is another. Motorists should not have to continue to pay with their lives to keep the trucks rolling in their present design condition and thus to save the owners and manufacturers a few dollars. There should be under run guards at passenger vehicle bumper height, and lights and reflectors, spaced widely, at 15 inches above the pavement, where they can be seen and localized on the roadway. Truck and trailer wheels should be better shielded to reduce road spray and dirt collection; mud guards as now used are only partially effective.

BLACK VS. WHITE TIRES

One possible improvement in visibility at very little if any cost would be the use of tires made of white rubber throughout. If this were done, the tire tread against the pavement would provide a gleaming white surface for easy seeing by the motorist as he approaches from the rear. Although the side walls would get dirty, they would be better reflectors than the current black tires now in use.

The benefits in increased visibility for all vehicles would be worthwhile, and especially for trucks. White tire treads would provide localization clues superior to anything we have available today, and their visibility would improve with adverse weather because of their self-cleaning properties.

(*Text continues on page 170.*)

TABLE 9-10 EQUIPMENT
MULTIPURPOSE PASSENGER VEHICLES, TRUCKS, TRAILERS, AND BUSES OF 80 OR MORE INCHES OVERALL WIDTH

Item	Number and color in accordance with Society of Automotive Engineers Standard J578a, April 1965 required on			In accordance with SAE Standard or Recommended Practice
	Multipurpose Passenger Vehicles, Trucks (other than Truck Tractors), and Buses	*Trailers*	*Truck Tractors*	
Head lamps	2 white, 7-inch, Type 2 head lamp units; or 2 white, 5¾-inch, Type 1 head lamp units and 2 white, 5¾-inch, Type 2 head lamp units	—	Same as trucks and buses	J580a, June 1966, and J579a, Aug. 1965
Tail lamps	2 red	2 red	2 red	J585c, June 1966
Stop lamps	2 red or amber	2 red or amber	2 red or amber	J586b, June 1966
License plate lamp	1 white	1 white	1 white	J587b, April 1964
Reflex reflectors	4 Class A red; 2 Class A amber	4 Class A red; 2 Class A amber	2 Class A red (on rear); 2 Class A amber	J594c, Feb. 1965
Side marker lamps	2 red; 2 amber	2 red; 2 amber	2 amber	J592b, April 1964
		—	1 white	J593b, May 1966

Device		2 Class A red or amber	2 Class A red or amber; 2 Class A amber	SAE Standard
Back-up lamp	1 white			J588d, June 1966
Turn signal lamps	2 Class A red or amber; 2 Class A amber			
Turn signal operating unit	1	—	1	J589, April 1964
Turn signal flasher	1	—	1	J590b, Oct. 1965
Vehicular hazard warning signal operating unit	1	—	1	J910, Jan. 1966
Vehicular hazard warning signal flasher	1	—	1	J945, Feb. 1966
Identification lamps	3 amber, and 3 red	3 red	3 amber	J592b, April 1964
Clearance lamps	2 amber and 2 red	2 amber and 2 red	2 amber	J592b, April 1964
Intermediate side marker lamps	2 amber	2 amber	—	J592b, April 1964
Intermediate reflex reflectors	2 Class A amber	2 Class A amber	—	J594c, Feb. 1965

TABLE 9-11 LOCATION OF EQUIPMENT

MULTIPURPOSE PASSENGER VEHICLES, TRUCKS, TRAILERS, AND BUSES OF 80 OR MORE INCHES OVERALL WIDTH

Item	Location on			Height above road surface measured from center of item on vehicle at curb weight
	Multipurpose Passenger Vehicles, Trucks (other than truck tractors), and Buses	Trailers	Truck Tractors	
Head lamps	Type 1 head lamps at the same height, 1 on each side of the vertical centerline; Type 2 head lamps at the same height, 1 on each side of the vertical centerline, as far apart as practicable	—	Same as trucks and buses	Not less than 24 inches nor more than 54 inches
Tail lamps	On the rear, 1 on each side of the vertical centerline, at the same level, and as far apart as practicable	On the rear, 1 on each side of the vertical centerline, at the same level, and as far apart as practicable	One the rear, 1 on each side of the vertical centerline, at the same level, and as far apart as practicable	Not less than 15 inches, nor more than 72 inches
Stop lamps	On the rear, 1 on each side of the vertical centerline, at the same level, and as far apart as practicable	On the rear, 1 on each side of the vertical centerline, at the same level, and as far apart as practicable	On the rear, 1 on each side of the vertical centerline, at the same level, and as far apart as practicable	Not less than 15 inches nor more than 72 inches
License plate lamp	At rear license plate	At rear license plate	At rear license plate	—
Reflex reflectors	2 red—on rear, 1 on each side of the vertical centerline, as far apart as practicable and at the same level	2 red—on rear, 1 on each side of the vertical centerline as far apart as practicable and at the same level.	2 red—on rear, 1 on each side of the vertical centerline, as far apart as practicable and at the same level (1)	Not less than 15 inches nor more than 60 inches

Item	Location on			Height above road surface measured from center of item on vehicle at curb weight
	Multipurpose Passenger Vehicles, Trucks (other than truck tractors), and Buses	Trailers	Truck Tractors	
	2 red—on sides, 1 on each side as far aft as practicable 2 amber—on sides 1 on each side as far forward as practicable	2 red—on sides, 1 on each side as far aft as practicable 2 amber—on sides, 1 on each side as far forward as practicable	2 amber—on sides, 1 on each side as far forward as practicable	Not less than 15 inches
Side marker lamps	*On each side:* 1 red lamp as far to the rear as practicable and 1 amber lamp as far forward as practicable.	*On each side:* 1 red lamp as far to the rear as practicable and 1 amber lamp as far forward as practicable	*On each side:* 1 amber lamp as far forward as practicable	—
Back-up lamp	On rear, so that the optical center of the lens surface is visible from any eye point elevation from 2 feet to 6 feet above the horizontal plane on which the vehicle is standing, and from any position in the area rearward of a vertical plane, perpendicular to the longitudinal axis of the vehicle 3 feet to the rear of the vehicle, and extending 3 feet beyond each side of the vehicle.	—	On rear, so that the optical center of the lens surface is visible from any eye point elevation from 2 feet to 6 feet above the horizontal plane on which the vehicle is standing, and from any position in the area rearward of a vertical plane, perpendicular to the longitudinal axis of the vehicle 3 feet to the rear of the vehicle, and extending 3 feet beyond each side of the vehicle	

TABLE 9-11 (CONTINUED)

Item	Multipurpose Passenger Vehicles, Trucks (other than truck tractors), and Buses	Location on Trailers	Truck Tractors	Height above road surface measured from center of item on vehicle at curb weight
Turn signal lamps	*At or near the front:* 1 amber on each side of the vertical centerline, at the same level, and as far apart as practicable. *On rear:* 1 red or amber on each side of the vertical centerline, at the same level, and as far apart as practicable	*On rear:* 1 red or amber on each side of the vertical centerline, at the same level, and as far apart as practicable	*At or near the front:* 1 amber on each side of the vertical centerline, at the same level, and as far apart as practicable. *On rear:* 1 red or amber on each side of the vertical centerline, at the same level, and as far apart as practicable	Not less than 15 inches
Identification lamps	*On front and rear:* 3 lamps, amber in front red in rear, grouped in a horizontal row, with lamp centers spaced not less than 6 inches, nor more than 12 inches, apart and mounted as close as practicable to the vertical centerline	*On rear:* 3 red lamps grouped in a horizontal row with lamp centers spaced not less than 6 inches, nor more than 12 inches, apart and mounted as close as practicable to the vertical centerline	*On front:* 3 amber lamps grouped in a horizontal row with lamp centers spaced not less than 6 inches, nor more than 12 inches, apart and mounted as close as practicable to the vertical centerline	*On front only:* No part of the lamps or mountings may extend below the top of the vehicle's windshield

Item	Location on — Multipurpose Passenger Vehicles, Trucks (other than truck tractors), and Buses	Location on — Trailers	Location on — Truck Tractors	Height above road surface measured from center of item on vehicle at curb weight
Clearance lamps	*On front and rear:* 1 amber lamp in front, 1 red lamp in rear, as near as practicable to the upper left and right extreme edges of the vehicle. When the rear identification lamps are mounted at the extreme height of the vehicle, rear clearance lamps may be mounted at optional heights	*On front and rear:* 1 amber lamp in front, 1 red lamp in rear, as near as practicable to the upper left and right extreme edges of the vehicle. When the rear identification lamps are mounted at the extreme height of the vehicle, rear clearance lamps may be mounted at optional heights	*On front:* 1 amber lamp as near as practicable to the upper left and right extreme edges of the vehicle	—
Intermediate side marker lamps	*On each side:* 1 amber lamp located at or near the midpoint between the forward and aft side marker lamps	*On each side:* 1 amber lamp located at or near the midpoint between the forward and aft side marker lamps	—	Not less than 15 inches
Intermediate side reflex reflectors	*On each side:* 1 amber located at or near the midpoint between the forward and aft side reflex reflectors	*On each side:* 1 amber located at or near the midpoint between the forward and aft side reflex reflectors	—	Not less than 15 inches nor more than 60 inches

ONE TO FOUR A.M.

The incidence of fatal one-car accidents is extremely high in the early morning hours. The confirmed explanation of this phenomenon is not at hand; however, a look at some of the factors is in order. First is the matter of fatigue and the need for sleep.

One should never drive after his normal bedtime, because about two hours after normal bedtime it becomes difficult if not impossible to stay awake. By about two o'clock in the morning one enters a sleep-producing driving environment. The traffic on the highway is sparse; therefore the bright points of light from tail and headlights are missing most of the time. All that remains is the dark of the night, with a gradual brightening in the lower field of view as the pavement comes nearer to the headlights. Neither vegetation nor the surface of the pavement can be clearly focused upon because of the low illumination and their steady "movement" as the automobile proceeds. Darkness allows pupil dilation, which tends to cause blurring due to aberrations. Darkness may also allow accommodation to increase, sometimes as much as 1.5 diopters, further blurring the limited detail available. The rapidly reducing strength of the visual stimulation because of increased blurring and lowered illumination is similar to that encountered with the eyes closed, when sleep readily occurs.

A hypnotic effect at night is undoubtedly involved; however, the distinction between a hypnotic trance and real sleep is difficult to make when a subject is unduly fatigued past his bedtime. Alcohol, carbon monoxide (cigarettes and automobile exhaust), and a full stomach are all predisposing factors. Each or all may team up with fatigue, the absence of detail in the roadway scene, and the hypnotic nature of the driving task to overcome even the best driver.

The loss of visual control is real. It appears that a nystagmus develops which lowers acuity. This is accompanied by a loss of fusion and an extreme urge to close the eyes. Such danger signs cannot be ignored! On the highway, one should open the window, turn up the radio, turn on the dome light, turn up the dash light, and indulge in singing and isometrics until he reaches the nearest stopping point.

The use of the interior lighting of the vehicle, including brightening the dash panel, is most comforting when driving for long periods at night. Fusion recovers, acuity improves, and the darkness seems literally to be pushed away when it had been in danger of engulfing the tired driver. The fear of destroying dark adaptation by having extra light in the car should be overbalanced by the fear of the complete loss of orientation which occurs with fatigue under low levels of illumination. Actually, dark adaptation to levels lower than the roadway will not occur, and normal interior lighting can have very little effect on the level of adaptation needed for the external scene. The only precaution is to be sure that the dash panel does not reflect into the windshield and that the windshield is clean. Observations indicate a very slight loss of visual range with interior lighting. At the same time vision seems clearer, probably due to a smaller pupil.

A number of ideas to add detail in the outside scene at night have been proposed. Small points of light on posts at the front edges of the hood would assure ocular focus and would help maintain vehicle and driver orientation. A bright reticle or cross hair, as used in military gun sights, could be optically projected into the roadway, perhaps off the windshield's back surface. Such a target would be excellent for maintaining convergence and accommodation under control. However, it would have to have a large aperture of perhaps 12 inches to permit freedom of head movement, and it would be both difficult to install and expensive to build. Nevertheless, plastic Fresnel lens components might provide the break-through needed.

The ultimate goal for night driving is more light. Both the Bridge side light and the proposed side lighting (see Figure 9-7) supply surround light with a noticeable increase in comfort. European driving lights, for example the Lucas quartz halogen lamp, supply such a remarkable increase in illumination that reticles and fender markers would probably become unnecessary.

Of course, the ideal admonition is to avoid driving during the early morning hours if one normally sleeps then. Avoid large meals, alcohol, and smoking (Adams and Belvin, 1966; MacFarland and Moseley, September 1954). Keep lights on bright as much as traffic will allow. If drowsiness seems to be occurring, change body position, change temperature in the car, turn on the radio and the dome light, and slow down 5 or 10 miles per hour; at least do not go faster "to get there sooner." If out of control of your body physiology, stop well off the pavement, at a service station, roadside park, or other protected location. If you stop along the highway, move at least ten feet off the pavement, turn off your headlights, set your emergency four-way flasher into operation, turn off your engine, and take a nap. The hazard of roadside stopping without the four-way flasher is that your normal red tail lights may lure another sleepy driver to follow you right off the pavement and collide with you. Above all, do not take a walk on the pavement, because few drivers will be looking out for a pedestrian. Even if they were, the chances are against the pedestrian being seen in time. If the shoulders are muddy, or the roadway is not wide enough to pull off at least ten feet, drive carefully until you find a service station or other safe location.

HEADLIGHT LAWS

A driver will have trouble seeing oncoming cars against the setting or rising sun, while oncoming drivers will be able to see perfectly well with the sun behind them. However, they should have their headlights on to help them to be seen. Many states require headlights to be turned on by thirty minutes after sunset to thirty minutes before sunrise. Such legislation should be changed to ensure that headlights must be turned on at least one hour *before* sunset and not turned off sooner than one hour *after* sunrise, if then. This would require headlights to be on any time the sun is lower than 15 degrees from the horizon. It is hoped that legislators would require headlights to be on all day long.

Certainly, the rule of headlights on thirty minutes after the sun sets and off thirty minutes before the sun rises is archaic and unrealistic for today's driving. Figure 9-10 indicates that motorists themselves find driving without lights after sunset unacceptable. The far north, as in Alaska, has a poorly defined sunset and prolonged poor seeing, hence a safer rule for all states is to have headlights on any time the engine is running. Since accidents are more frequent in the late afternoon hours and since this time is very difficult for drivers, especially on two-lane free access roads and highways, the motorist would be wise to stop and have a light supper and, if necessary, continue the trip after the sun has set.

DAYTIME HAZARDS

SUN AND SKY GLARE

On a bright sunny day who would think visibility could be a problem? Yet, as discussed in Chapters 2 and 8, numerous factors degrade vision in the daytime. Accident statistics show clear dry days to be especially hazardous. The most disabling circumstance in the daytime occurs when the sun is in the driver's forward field of view. The nearer it is to the line of sight of the driver, the more disabling. The eye becomes adapted to the high luminance levels. It is hampered by the stray light in the eye and the fact that all hazardous objects on the ground are viewed from their dark or shadowed side. Polished concrete or asphalt pavement may gleam like a ribbon of fire from a low-hanging sun. Seeing people, cars, or even trucks becomes impossible under certain situations and difficult under virtually all situations with a low sun. Nonpolarizing sunglasses make the seeing situation against the sun worse because they reduce the visibility of the already inadequately lighted objects in the field of view. Polarizing sunglasses will reduce pavement glare and windshield reflections and may improve vision.

Sky glare and sun glare usually are efficiently controlled with the sun visor provided in most cars. This has proven to be the most useful device in glare experiments for improving visual performance. Among the many sources of glare, sky glare seems to be as serious or more serious than any other. Reflection from the top of the hood can be distressing if the hood is of light color and highly polished. There is a new transparent paint which removes the gloss without changing the appearance of the automobile paint.* It should prove popular, especially among police and fleet owners.

Reflections from the top of the dash panel off the back side of the windshield are still excessive in some new automobiles. As mentioned before, an adequate solution is a piece of black velveteen draped over the top of the dash. Dirt on the windshield or on spectacles provides an amount of glare proportional to the amount of dirt and direction of the sun. The solution is to clean the spectacles and operate the windshield washer.

ATMOSPHERIC BOIL

This condition is seen on hot days as a shimmering and unsteadiness of objects at a great distance. The effect is due to shifting of the optical density of the air due to wind and temperature differences. This phenomenon reduces the visual acuity for objects seen outdoors through several hundred feet of atmosphere compared to clinical acuity. The reduction in acuity depends upon the amount of atmosphere between the eyes and the target and the thermal discontinuities in the atmosphere. Under most conditions where highway signs are involved, acuity should not fall very much. However, conditions can vary widely in the atmosphere, and if one needs to know the acuity possible in a given circumstance, his best approach is to measure it. Atmospheric boil is at a minimum right after sunrise and just before sunset. It is maximum when the solar radiation is greatest. It is at a constant second maximum during the night hours. The effect is present winter or summer and is least on overcast days.

Atmospheric attenuation and sky light also tend to reduce the contrast of distant objects; hence for optimum visibility a sign or an object must have a high contrast with its background. With increasing speeds we need some signs to be legible from 2,000 feet or more. Certainly, this kind of visibility cannot be provided in every kind of weather, no matter how big we make the sign. The freeway sign that slips by in the fog without being seen in time to read it is a case in point.

Thus, it seems that a series of advance warning information signs in addition to the main sign are imperative to ensure that the motorist is informed of decisions to be made or actions to take. Visibility through short sections of the atmosphere will always be superior to that through longer sections, and perhaps the ideal sign system would be that placed nearby on the pavement itself. Color coding of lanes or of lane marking paint stripes has been shown to be of great value, at least in the daytime. Reflectorized colors would be necessary at night to permit enough light to be returned to the eyes to make the coloring effective.

* B Sure Representatives Inc., 1204 North Woodward, Royal Oak, Michigan 48067.

MIRAGE EFFECTS

Mirages occur regularly on the highways. While typically seen in the daytime as shimmering white light resembling water on the distant pavement surface, mirages also are seen for several hours after sunset. Then they behave like a base-up prism, refracting part of the rays from oncoming headlights to make them appear double as if two cars were approaching, one above the other. In the early morning hours, after the pavement has cooled more than the air, the surface air works like a base-down prism, bending light downward, thus somewhat increasing visibility over hills.

Probably the most significant hazard from daytime mirages is the delayed appearance of a vehicle approaching on the crest of a hill. The heated air near the pavement surface bends light upward so that the rays of light from an oncoming automobile do not travel in a straight line. Hence the automobile beyond the crest of a hill must come closer, to rise high enough, so that the bent light rays from it will arrive at our eyes, instead of going over our heads.

The heated air near the pavement also causes distant vehicles to disappear or to be so poorly defined that they cannot be accurately located or judged for speed. Sometimes a vehicle may be completely covered over by the bright sky light appearing to come from the boundary layer of air over the pavement. Others may lose some of their parts, such as their lower half or a portion in the middle.

Since the mirage of water on the highway is really a refracted image of the sky, a most unbearable glare from the pavement occurs when the part of the sky seen on the roadway contains the sun! Such a situation cannot be remedied effectively by any sunglasses, and the luminance level may become so high that the motorist will be forced, in the interest of safety, to pull into a rest area and wait fifteen or twenty minutes until the condition subsides before continuing to drive.

CAMOUFLAGE EFFECTS

The difference in luminance between an object and its background is a clue to an excellent camouflage technique. The smaller the luminance difference between an object and its background, the less likely will be the detection of the object. For example, when viewed from the air at low altitude, the highways are full of cars. As altitude increases, fewer cars are seen and they are the lighter colored ones only. The lightest colors are the last to disappear at very great altitude. When earth scenery is viewed from a car, its average luminance is about the same as a well-worn highway. Against this average background, measurements with a Luckiesh-Moss Visibility Meter show that light-colored automobiles are significantly more visible. Thus, gray- or dark-colored automobiles have an element of camouflage built in. The fact that 21-candle power running lights or 4-candle power parking lights reduce the number and the severity of accidents proves that such camouflage effects really do exist and do contribute to accidents.

A spotted Dalmatian dog sitting in the spotty shade of a tree will be camouflaged. This illustrates a second principle in camouflage: namely, the characteristic shape of an object can be disguised by adding meaningless spots, areas, and lines that could easily be confused with the background. Measurements on aircraft visibility both in the air and on the surface of the earth have shown that when an airplane was a single solid color it was the most detectable. When various patterns were used, the detectability was reduced in proportion to the amount of variegation, even for uniform sky viewing. Thus, two-tone paint patterns on automobiles are likely to be less visible than a single color, especially a light one. Automobile surfaces are already composed in large part of glass, which has, on the average, about the same luminance as the background. The popular black vinyl top, used with all conceivable paint colors, adds to the two-toning effect provided by the windows and is not a wise color choice because of a reduction in the visibility of the car and an increase in the heat uptake inside the car in the summer.

Chromium reflects about 50 percent of the light falling on it. Because it is usually highly polished, it sparkles and brightly images the sun. Under many conditions the reflections from chromium make a car very visible. However, since chromium behaves like a mirror, there may be reflections from dark-colored objects at a given moment, whereupon the chromium looks dark or even black. Chromium therefore cannot be relied upon to provide the visibility that a dark-colored automobile needs. On the other hand, bright metal surfaces on one's own car that reflect the sun tend to interfere with vision and to increase the effectiveness of camouflage on streets and highways.

The most effective technique is to hide the object rather than to disguise it. The automobile discovered in front of the truck one is passing was hidden from view. An automobile in a fog is hidden. The pedestrian or automobile partially or completely covered by the windshield corner posts or the rear-view mirror is hidden. Even the dirt spots on the windshield and the dangling toys in some cars will hide or partially obscure an object on a collision course. This is true because an object on a collision course does not change its position in the field of view of the driver, although it does get larger. Since objects attached to the car, such as windshield dirt spots, do not change their position either, they interfere with a view of the outside object. Hiding tail and headlights from oblique view by forward and rearward jutting fenders led the government to require reflectors and/or side marker lights beginning with the 1968 models. Darkness is itself great camouflage.

Modern styling is used to modify the estimate of speed and direction of an object. This is done by strong slanting lines added to confuse the real size and shape of an object. Styling has thinned the roof line, which reduces the apparent height of a passenger automobile and makes it appear farther away and thus to be going slower. Window, fender, and grill lines are slanted in various directions to give the illusion of motion. The prevalence in accident reports of the statement, "I didn't see—," indicates the effectiveness with which camouflage operates in driving a motor vehicle.

RAIN, MIST, SNOW, AND FOG

Daytime rain, mist, snow, and fog serve to reduce the contrast of objects seen from a motor vehicle, and thus they increase the already existing effects described above. Windshield dirt and water droplets tend to increase the detrimental effects occurring during rain due to the absence of shadows, atmospheric scattering, and dirt on roadway objects.

An especially significant hazard in adverse weather is the pedestrian. When getting wet, a human being becomes preoccupied. He will cover his head and run across a street or walk in front of an automobile. Pedestrians seem to picture the motorist as an inconsiderate person, sitting dry and comfortable in his car, watching the poor pedestrian getting wet. The pedestrian believes the motorist can see him, can stop, and will stop if there is any question about the pedestrian getting hurt. The motorist on the other hand has his own problems. The windshield wipers do not sweep all of the windshield area; the vision through what is wiped is not good; side windows, rear windows, and major parts of the windshield often are fogged. The motorist feels closed in. Because traffic moves slowly, he may become annoyed. Because pedestrians are taking unusual risks, he may feel that they are being "pushy" and are imposing upon him when he has so many other problems, many of them due to the weather. The confusion and poor visibility may be so adverse that he may not even see the pedestrian and he may be unfortunate enough to strike one.

Under adverse weather conditions it is imperative that vehicles have their lights on so that pedestrians and motorists can see them. Umbrellas should be transparent so the pedestrian can see approaching automobiles. Each person must be taught that he himself, in the final analysis, is the only person to be depended upon for personal safety. He must be convinced of the difficulties of being seen so he can act intelligently and safely. He must be made to understand that hair, hats, glasses, clothing, and anything else that interfere with side vision can cost him his life.

Chapter 10: Desirable Practices

STREET LIGHTING AS A SUPPLEMENT
TO HEADLIGHTING

NUMEROUS before and after studies in the United States have shown that increasing street illumination levels generally reduces accidents. Similar reductions in accidents have been observed in industry among factory workers. Few studies have been made of the effect on accidents of raising the highway illumination level by means of headlights alone. In England and Europe it is common practice to drive without headlights because an extensive system of street lighting exists. Studies in England requiring motorists to change traditional "parking lights," as we would call them, to low-beam headlights in the city produced conflicting results, due partly at least to partial compliance and the mixing of the two types of lighting. Parking-lighted automobiles mixed with head-lighted automobiles puts the parking-lighted automobile at a serious disadvantage in overall visibility. A similar difficulty arises in the daytime between automobiles using headlights and those not using headlights. In states where holiday "lights-on" campaigns have been held, more than half of the motorists failed to cooperate. Hence mass statistics do not clearly support the thesis that daytime headlights increase safety and they may actually increase the hazard to the driver who fails to participate.

There is a conflict between headlighting and street lighting such that a pedestrian, seen in silhouette by light reflected off the polished pavement from the overhead lights beyond him, will lose some of his visibility at a critical distance from the automobile headlights. At this point clothing blends into the background pavement. This could only occur within a limited zone in front of the automobile, depending upon the reflectance of the clothing, the aim of the headlights, and the intensity of street light reflected from the roadway. Also, since pedestrians are rela-

177

tively tall compared to automobile headlights and since the headlight distribution varies with elevation above the road, especially on low beams, it is unlikely that all of the pedestrian will be invisible at once. Only a part of the pedestrian would be of the same luminance as the pavement, the parts above being darker and the parts below being brighter than the background pavement. The lower the intensity of the street lighting and headlighting, the more serious becomes the tendency for the headlights and street lights to cancel one another at certain distances. Conversely, the higher the levels of illumination, the more efficient is the eye and the better will be the visual performance.

For those who would emphasize street lighting and exclude automobile headlighting, it is well to keep in mind that even full daytime natural street lighting shows an additional reduction in accidents when headlights and other running lights are used. We need both types of lighting and as much of both as we can afford. There is no one best way to light our highways and streets!

Street lighting is most efficient for seeing something on the pavement when it provides silhouette lighting, but objects off the pavement would probably not be seen with such lighting. To solve this the Texas Transportation Institute has been experimenting with 150-foot-high artificial moonlight sources which have been used as street lighting in Austin, Texas, since 1894. Large clusters of lamps with direction-controlling reflectors are mounted on poles 200 to 300 feet high (see Figure 10-1) near cloverleaf interchanges on important highways. They report both economy in installation and better seeing. The overall effect is comfortable because one can see the highway and the lighted countryside without the feeling of confinement by the limits of the headlight pattern. Low (10- to 30-inch) street lighting with no upward component has met with considerable acceptance in fog. The lights are directed across the road from either side and have been used, for example, on a number of new bridges as a designed-in feature.

EDGE AND CENTER-LINE MARKINGS

Studies have shown that pavement markings are among the most effective means of controlling traffic flow and imparting information to the driver. Marking the edge of the pavement causes the traffic to move away from the edge. This is beneficial because dropping a wheel off the edge of the pavement is a frequent cause of being forcefully redirected across the road into oncoming traffic or into a skidding or overturn accident. Center-line marking serves to stabilize traffic at a safer distance away from the center as well. Reflectorization of these lines with beaded

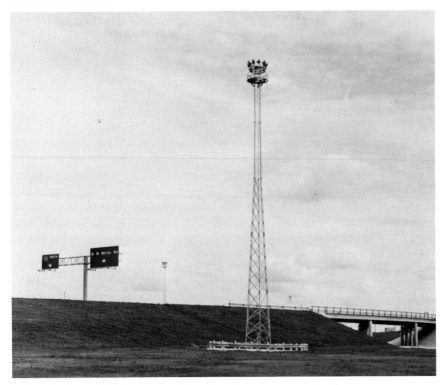

Figure 10-1. Tower lighting for freeway interchange. Second tower can be seen to the left beyond the highway. A third tower can be seen just to the right of the main tower and still farther away. Note that guard rails are used around the base of the tower to reduce the likelihood of a fatal crash into the tower structure. (Photograph supplied by the Texas Transportation Institute, Texas A & M College.)

paint is a significant help at night. "Cat's eye" surface-adhering retro-reflectors * serve about the same purpose as reflectorized paint and they are more rainproof. However, snowplows destroy them within a single winter; hence their use is confined to southern states at the present time. Should the snowplow problem be solved by a change over to plastic or rubber plow blades or by an improved plow-resistant reflector design, the waterproof reflectors should be put into more widespread use, because they are needed in adverse weather. It is possible to improve the performance of beaded paints in rain; however, even cat's eye units become useless if water inundates them as on a poorly drained road.

* A retroreflector composed of one or more optical elements of about one half inch across. The essential feature is that it returns light much as does a cat's eye.

REFLECTORIZATION

Reflectorization of hazards at night serves to increase their visibility by making more efficient use of available light. Reflectorization is desirable for pavement paint, license plates, highway safety signs, street signs, pedestrians, bicycles, slow-moving vehicles, trucks, trains, buses, and automobiles. Reflectorization of fence posts, driveways, business signs, and so on is not desirable. Reflectors must be functional; that is, they must locate and identify an obstacle, sign, or edge of the highway. They must not appear to hang in space, seemingly unattached to the ground or to an object. A pedestrian carrying a dangling reflector or reflectors attached to his shoes or clothes may be identified as a pedestrian by the motion of the reflector as he walks; but if he stands still, the reflections might be construed to be from a fence post, a cat, or even a discarded can.

Outline reflectorization of motorcycles, bicycles, buses, trucks, or trains clarifies the nature of the hazard, where it is, and how fast it is being overtaken. In an ocean of point reflectors, as might exist ten years from now, the driver would be easily confused by the possible chaos. If substance is added by changing points to outlines that tie together the lights and point reflectors, order returns out of confusion. Thus wide-spaced tail lights may not appear to be on the same vehicle unless joined together by some structure that is lighted or reflectorized. Ford Motor Company has placed strips of reflectorized material along the sides of certain sporty production models, and the 3M Company has developed a reflectorized sidewall material for tires. Both serve the purpose of location and identification, especially when used together. It is hoped that greater use of sheet reflective materials on tires and other parts of trucks, buses, motorcycles, bicycles, passenger cars—and on pedestrians—will develop in the near future. Quicker detection, localization, and identification will be the assured result.

FLUORESCENT MATERIALS

Fluorescence is the physical process by which short-wavelength high-energy radiations are absorbed and re-radiated at a longer wavelength. The outdoor environment at sunset and twilight contains mostly the shorter, relatively invisible solar radiations. Fluorescent materials (including those in laundry detergents) convert this energy into light in the visible spectrum. Objects coated with such materials reflect the ordinary amounts of visible light plus the visible light produced by converting the

(*Text continues on page 197.*)

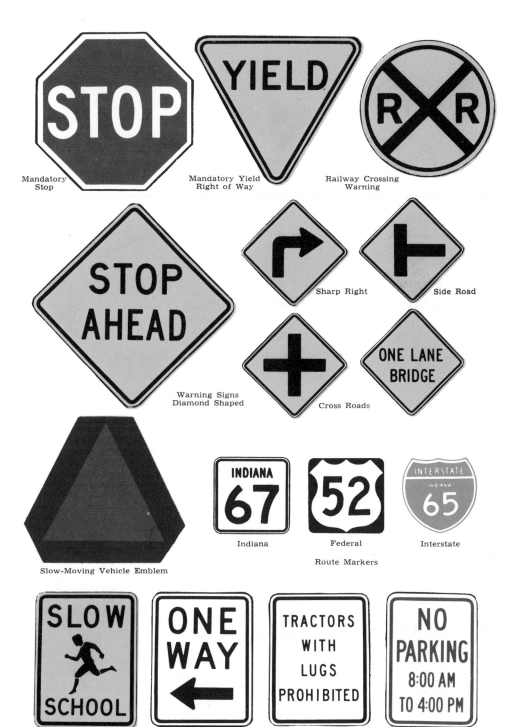

Figure 10-2. Principal signs used on highways in the United States of America. Relative sizes in this figure are of no importance. Local conditions, traffic speed, and legislative requirements determine the sizes in actual use.

181

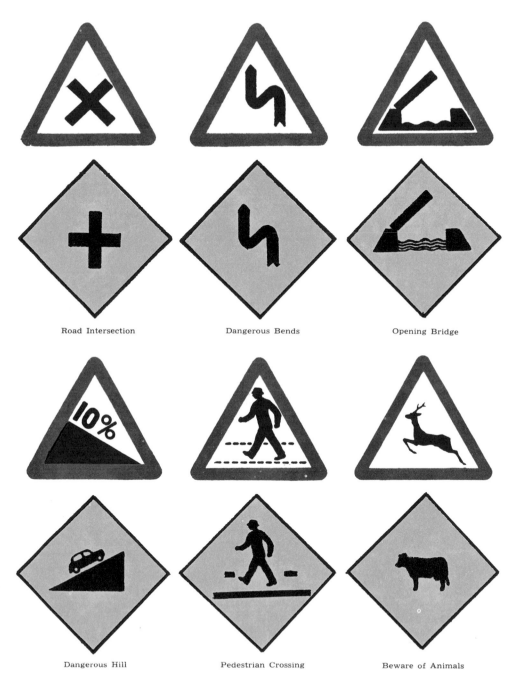

Road Intersection Dangerous Bends Opening Bridge

Dangerous Hill Pedestrian Crossing Beware of Animals

Figure 10-3. United Nations motorway warning signs. The red triangle, apex up, is interchangeable with the yellow diamond for all warning signs.

182

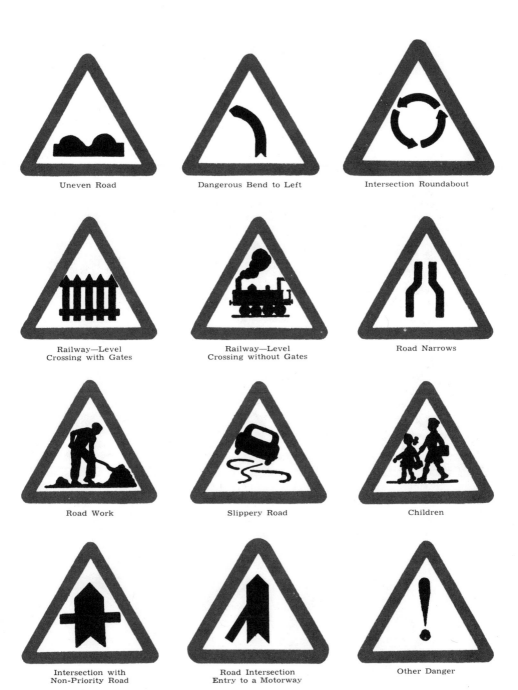

Figure 10-4. United Nations motorway warning signs. The black figures may also be displayed on a yellow diamond background.

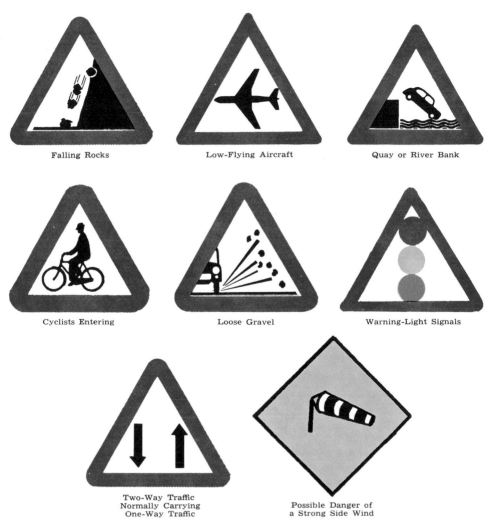

Figure 10-5. United Nations motorway warning signs. The yellow diamond or red triangle are optional backgrounds.

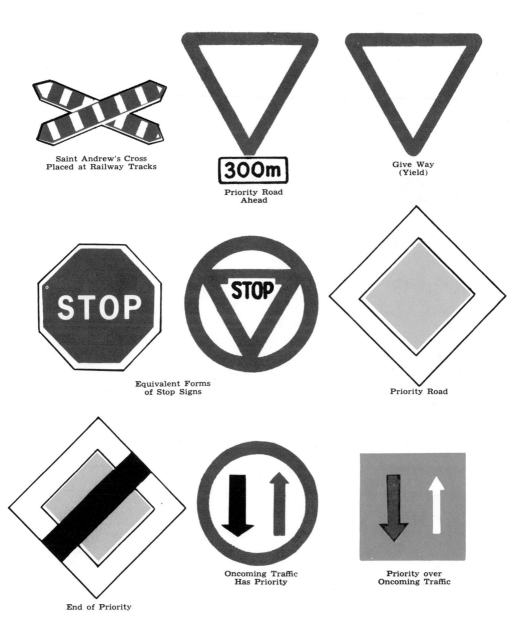

Saint Andrew's Cross
Placed at Railway Tracks

300m

Priority Road
Ahead

Give Way
(Yield)

STOP

Equivalent Forms
of Stop Signs

Priority Road

End of Priority

Oncoming Traffic
Has Priority

Priority over
Oncoming Traffic

Figure 10-6.   United Nations motorway mandatory signs. The red triangle displayed apex downward is not interchangeable with a yellow diamond except as shown here.

185

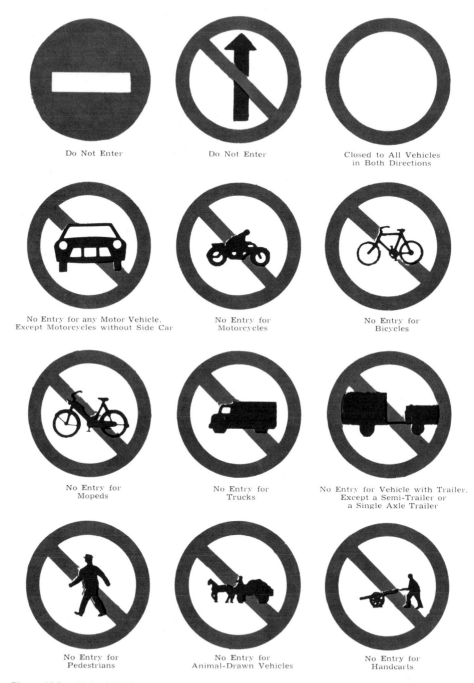

Figure 10-7. United Nations motorway prohibitory signs. The red circle signifies negative action; the black figure signifies the act or vehicle that is negated.

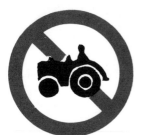

No Entry for Powered
Agricultural Vehicles

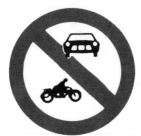

No Entry for
Power Driven Vehicles

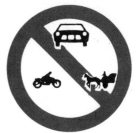

No Entry for
Power Driven Vehicles
or Animal-Drawn Vehicles

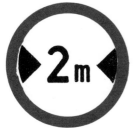

No Entry for Vehicles
Wider than 2 Meters

No Entry for Vehicles
Higher than 3.5 Meters

No Entry for Vehicles
over 5 Tons Loaded

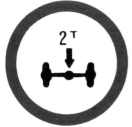

No Entry for Vehicles
over 2 Tons on One Axle

No Entry for Vehicles
or Combinations
Longer than 10 Meters

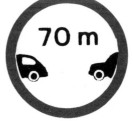

Vehicle Spacing Less
than 70 Meters Prohibited

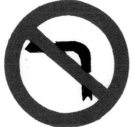

No Left Turn

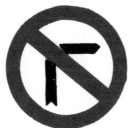

No Right Turn

No U-Turns

Figure 10-8.   United Nations motorway prohibitory signs (continued).

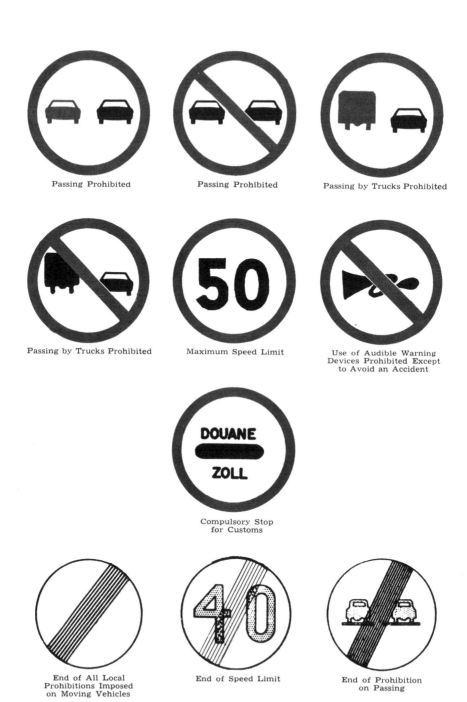

Figure 10-9. United Nations motorway prohibitory signs (continued). Note the black and white circular signs that signify the end of the prohibition imposed earlier.

188

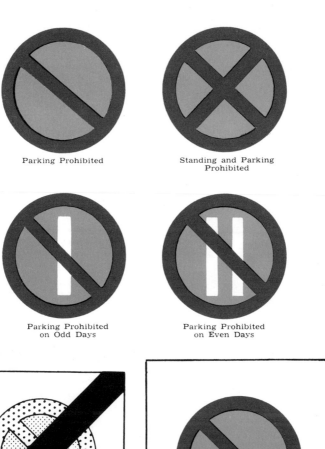

Parking Prohibited

Standing and Parking
Prohibited

Parking Prohibited
on Odd Days

Parking Prohibited
on Even Days

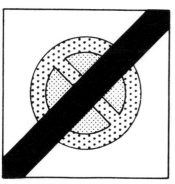

Exit Limited Duration
Parking Zone

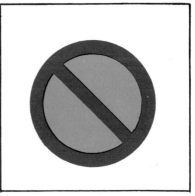

Limited Duration Parking Zone

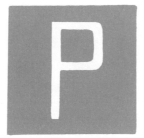

Parking Permitted

Figure 10-10.   United Nations parking regulatory signs.

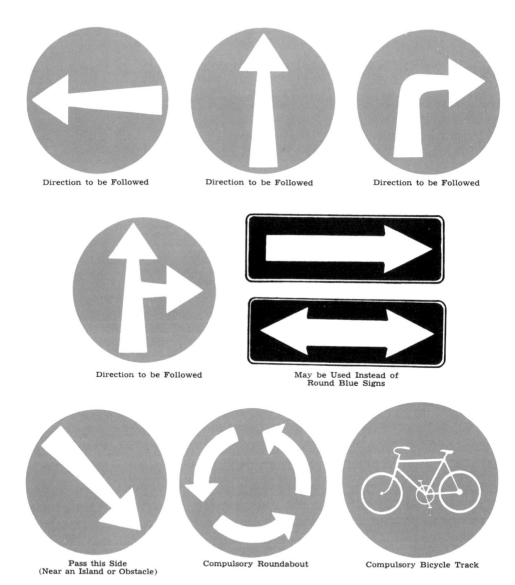

Direction to be Followed

Direction to be Followed

Direction to be Followed

Direction to be Followed

May be Used Instead of
Round Blue Signs

Pass this Side
(Near an Island or Obstacle)

Compulsory Roundabout

Compulsory Bicycle Track

Figure 10-11.   Examples of United Nations motorway compulsory signs. A blue circular sign is used with enclosed pattern to signify directions to be taken.

190

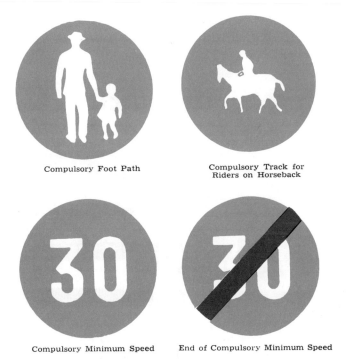

Compulsory Foot Path

Compulsory Track for
Riders on Horseback

Compulsory Minimum Speed

End of Compulsory Minimum Speed

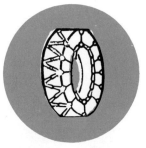

Snow Chains Compulsory

Figure 10-12.   Examples of United Nations motorway compulsory signs (continued).

191

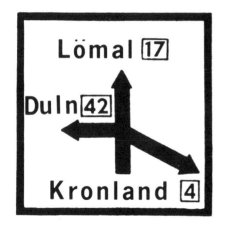

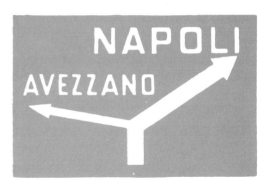

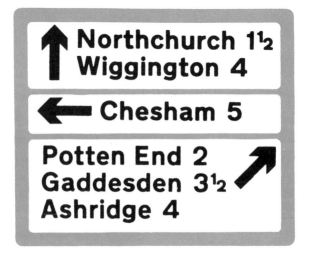

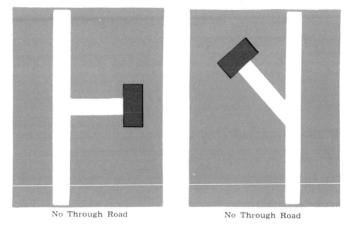

No Through Road No Through Road

Figure 10-13. Examples of United Nations motorway advanced direction and information signs.

192

GENÈVE

Entering Genève

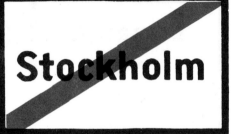

Leaving Stockholm

Direction to Tejerias Airport ← **TEJERIAS** ✈

🌲🏠 **500 m** Direction to a Youth Hostel

Direction to Lyon Airport **LYON** ✈

GENÈVE 17 Km Direction to Genève

Direction to Stockholm **17 Stockholm** **15**

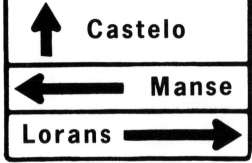

Directions to Castelo, Manse and Lorans

Héréra	2^{km}
SAN JOSE	35^{km}

Confirmatory Sign

Figure 10-14.   Examples of United Nations motorway direction signs. The city or township limits are indicated by the larger rectangular white or blue signs.

193

Pedestrian Crosswalk

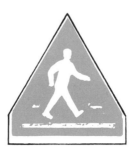

Pedestrian Crosswalk

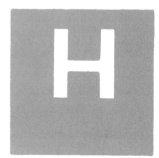

Hospital

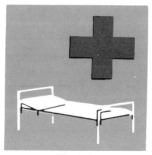

Hospital

One-Way Road

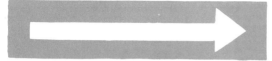

One-Way Sign Placed Parallel to Traffic

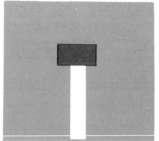

No Through Road

Figure 10-15.   Examples of United Nations motorway information signs.

194

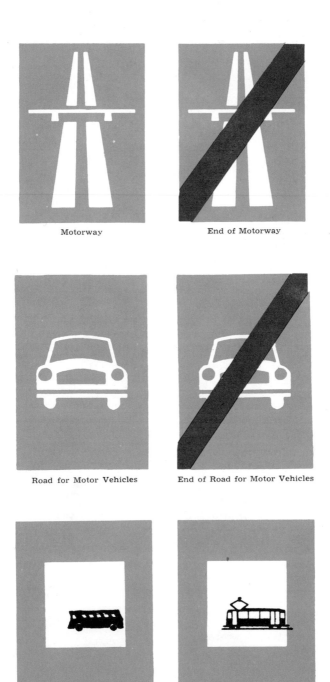

Figure 10-16. Examples of United Nations motorway information signs (continued).

195

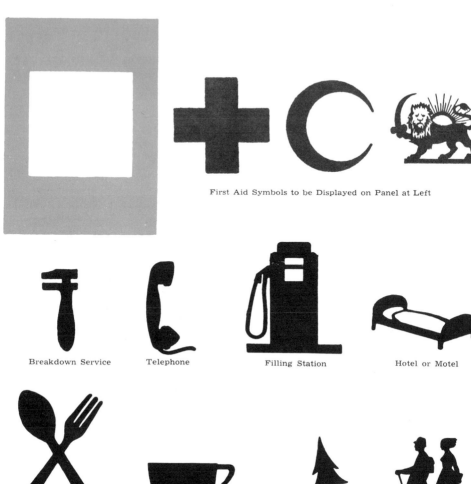

First Aid Symbols to be Displayed on Panel at Left

Breakdown Service

Telephone

Filling Station

Hotel or Motel

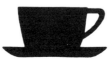

Restaurant

Refreshments or Cafeteria

Picnic Site

Starting Point for Walks

Camping Site

Caravan Site

Camping and
Caravan Site

Youth Hostel

Figure 10-17. Examples of United Nations motorway information signs (continued). The blue rectangle with white center may be displayed with any of the black or red figures shown. The red symbols are of special importance because each signifies First Aid.

shorter wavelength energy received. By choosing fluorescent materials that radiate energy at or near 555 nanometers, the peak sensitivity wavelength for the eye in the daytime, a remarkable brightness increase is possible. It has been found that an orange color is most attention-getting at dusk, partly because of color contrast and partly because the performance of the fluorescent materials currently available is better in this region.

At night fluorescent colors are without value because there is no available energy to operate them. However, some mercury arc and fluorescent artificial light installations may activate them. In the daytime the fluorescence phenomenon occurs at such a high intensity and temperature that chemical bonds are broken and the life of the material is greatly reduced. Even the more durable materials used on school zone signs, school buses, and slow-moving vehicle signs, for example, have a useful life of no more than three years, losing about 50 percent of their brightness per year.

Fluorescent materials are excellent hazard markers when visibility otherwise is extremely adverse, namely on dreary days and in late afternoon, early morning, and during twilight on clear days. As a warning of highway construction and other hazards, new fluorescent plastic flags have been observed to be significantly brighter than red signal lights and are detectable up to a mile away in the daytime.

School zone signs using fluorescent materials are easily spotted and read, especially under adverse weather conditions. Since the fluorescent layer is applied over a white base coat, deterioration of such signs with exposure to weather and ultraviolet light causes a lightening in color, usually to nonfluorescent yellow, which is similar to normal signs in visibility. Thus, it is safe to use florescent materials on such signs, even though their effectiveness slowly reduces back to that of a nonfluorescent normal sign.

VEHICLE VISIBILITY

A school bus that has a six-inch stripe of fluorescent material outlining it on the front, rear, and sides will have an added degree of conspicuousness which is needed when stops are made on the highway, especially during adverse weather. By outlining the bus, identification is assured, and the rate of overtake on the highway can be judged more accurately.

Police, fire, and ambulance vehicles need to be as conspicuous as possible. No doubt can exist about their daytime conspicuousness when they are coated with fluorescent material or about seeing them at night when outline-reflectorized. Emergency vehicles need to be as large as possible to make their speed and direction of movement apparent. Outlining probably is almost as effective as solid coverage with fluorescent and reflectorized material. A far less effective use of fluorescent material would be to spot it here and there, which, in effect, would camouflage it.

A motorcycle has such a small frontal area that a headlight is now required to be displayed at all times in some states to ensure that it will be seen. The tail light on the rear is a help in adverse weather but inadequate on a bright day. The lateral area of the machine should be protected by fluorescent materials as well as by reflectorized material. The cyclist himself needs both fluorescent and reflective materials on his helmet, jacket, and trousers to ensure visibility from all directions.

A bicycle is a low-visibility object of great vulnerability. Its proneness to accidents is increased because cyclists often ignore stop signs and other traffic rules. They are handicapped because of their poor maneuverability and by lack of adequate structure to provide a good visual target. At night significant visibility is provided if the frame, fenders, and wheel rims are reflectorized. The rider himself must also wear reflectorized materials, the more the better. In the daytime a bicycle headlight comparable to that of a motorcycle would be of assistance but is not available; hence fluorescent materials worn by the cyclist himself are the best protection. A waistband, jacket, or other fluorescent clothing is highly desirable for all bicycle riders.

Bike riders should be encouraged to stay on the sidewalks as much as possible. Although most sidewalks stand idle, bicyclists are prohibited by law in most states from riding on them. The most effective way to prevent cyclist-automobile accidents is to remove the cyclist from the streets. In Europe virtually every highway or road has a paved bicycle path paralleling it at a safe distance. There the pedestrians, bicycles, and motorized bicycles can mingle with much greater safety than on the highway itself. In the cities and towns, separate cycle paths as well as sidewalks often parallel the streets.

For trains a fluorescent panel at least one foot square, placed every ten feet along the sides of each car, would be helpful in preventing daytime side crash accidents. While these accidents are not frequent, 786 in 1967 (U.S. Department of Transportation, 1968), they still account for two thirds as many as the nighttime side-impact accidents of highway vehicles into trains. In the daytime, highway traffic is four times greater than at night, while railway traffic is the same as at night. Since only two thirds as many side-impact accidents happen between car and train in the daytime, one may conclude that trains are considerably less visible at night than they are in the daytime. In the daytime the train runs into the automobile three times as often as the automobile runs into the side of the train. At night, the automobile runs into the side of the train about 3 percent more frequently. Nighttime as well as daytime visibility of the locomotive is apparently inadequate. The high-placed headlight of the locomotive at night seems not to make it more visible. Outlining the locomotive both front and side with 12-inch-wide fluorescent strips should reduce the number of daytime accidents of the type where people do not see the train as they run into its path. Extrapolation from experiences with running lights indicates that between a 35 percent and 50 percent reduction in daytime train accidents would occur if the entire train were protected with fluorescent materials and if lights were displayed on the locomotive in the daytime as well as at night.

Protective headlighting for a locomotive of two 7-inch automobile Type Two headlights,* mounted low on the outer extremities at the forward end of the locomotive and aimed forward, would provide useful clues to the judgment of distance and speed of a train. In addition two 7-inch Type Two automobile headlights should be mounted to direct their beams horizontally at 45 and 90 degrees to the right and left of the direction of travel on each side of the locomotive. All six headlights should be flashed from low to high and back again constantly at a speed of about one cycle every two seconds. These lights and the main headlight of the locomotive should be on at any time of the night or day that the train is in operation and when it obstructs a crossing.

HIGHWAY SIGNS

Much study has been directed toward the best way to give a driver information about hazards and routes. The American system of signs has been under study for a considerable time and improvements have been made (Forbes et al., 1968). There are indications that still further improvements are needed. Figure 10-2 shows the principle highway signs as detailed in the 1969 Indiana Driver's Licensing Information Manual. It can be seen that there are five principal types of signs: round for railroad, octagonal for stop, diamond for hazard warning, triangular for yield, and rectangular for information.

It is apparent from various researches that for distinctiveness the octagonal and circular signs are the poorest, while the triangular and long rectangular shapes are the best. Information is also at hand to indicate that reliance on the red color of stop signs is foolhardy because of the low visibility of painted red signs in the external scene and because of protanopic and protanomalous color-defective persons who drive. The only reliable thing left is the word STOP, which we hope can be read by everyone if it is large enough.

---

* Type Two headlights have both high- and low-beam filaments.

In Europe the difficulty of a multiplicity of languages has led to the development of a pictorial sign system. The signs presented here represent the majority of signs used in Europe and elsewhere. The European system is based on the Protocol on Road Signs and Signals as agreed upon by the United Nations Conference on Road and Motor Transports in Geneva in 1949 and revised in Vienna in 1968 (United Nations 1969). There are three classes of signs: danger warning, regulatory, and informative. Figures 10-3, 10-4, and 10-5 illustrate most of the danger signs. Note the use of the very distinctive triangular shape and the optional diamond shape.

Regulatory signs are divided into priority, prohibitory, and mandatory (see Figures 10-6 through 10-11). Priority signs have a variety of shapes including the standard American railroad crossing sign. Prohibitory signs are round with a red rim and a white center in which various instruction symbols are displayed. All such signs should be taken as negative; i.e., no entry, no speed greater than___, no turn, no pedestrians.

Mandatory signs are circular and blue in color, as indicated in Figure 10-11.

Signs that give information are rectangular in shape. They usually are blue in color with a white and black picture included in the center. If red is used, it must not be the predominant color. Figures 10-12 through 10-18 give examples of important information signs.

Chapter 11: Some Popular Misconceptions

SUNGLASSES

GLARE and sunglasses are inseparably associated in the public mind, even to the extent that occasionally a person will try to use sunglasses for night driving to reduce headlight glare. In one fatal accident the driver was slated for trial on manslaughter charges because it was believed he should have seen a child running to catch a school bus. The children and the driver of the school bus could see him clearly, and he was wearing sunglasses! He was driving against the morning sun, which was about 10 degrees above the horizon and directly above the shiny road. In addition to the sun and bright sky he faced 25,000 foot-lamberts of pavement brightness. The child, running from the deep shadows among a long row of mailboxes under large trees on the right, probably could not have been seen until she stepped out onto the shiny pavement. The driver would have seen better without the sunglasses, although in this case the conditions were so severe it is doubtful if the driver could have avoided hitting the child even if he had not been wearing sunglasses. For example, the flashing red school bus warning lights at the top of the bus were adjacent to the silver bus top, which was reflecting high-intensity sunlight at grazing incidence toward the driver, so he probably could not have seen the red lights. Furthermore the school bus was in front of two 75-foot-long house trailers and two tractor trailer trucks, a rather effective means of camouflaging the bus.

Some people believe that camouflage does not occur on the highway because they have never seen it. If the driver in the above example had not struck the child, whom he said he did not see until after the impact, he would never have recognized that she was there! She was camouflaged by veiling glare from bright sources and by standing among mailboxes. Many times a passenger will comment about some event on or along the roadway that the driver has failed to see. Perhaps it was behind a corner post, or adjacent to hood or chromium glare, or his attention was directed to another point in the scene. Often even after being directed to the object or event, a driver cannot find it. Thus it is easy to understand that many things—in fact, most things are camouflaged and not seen at all, or perhaps seen only after months of traveling the same route.

Sunglasses transmit less useful light as well as less glare, and when useful light levels are reduced to about 400 foot-lamberts, vision is optimum because of an increase in visual efficiency. When the sunglasses reduce critical objects significantly below this level, seeing is impaired. Hence seeing detail under shade trees is greatly improved by removal of sunglasses, especially when standing in the sun. The light from the back surface of the lenses reflected mostly from the face is more noticeable when useful light coming through the lenses is low. Dirt on the lens surfaces further reduces seeing performance for less bright objects.

The quality of ready-made sunglasses often is not ideal, being degraded by irregular refraction due to poor surface quality. Many are made of plastic whose durability is greatly inferior to glass and whose performance can be expected to deteriorate the very first time they are cleaned or wiped off. Comparison between clean glass and clean plexiglass windshields, as carefully maintained in military aircraft, shows that twice the loss in visual range occurs when looking through the plexiglass compared to the plate glass. The implications clearly do not favor plastic sunglasses, which usually are softer and scratch more easily than plexiglass.

TINTED WINDSHIELDS

The tinted windshield controversy has at present been won by the manufacturers, who in some automobiles are supplying 100 percent of their passenger vehicles with this extra-cost item. The controversy has been between those who claim that tint impairs night seeing and those who argue that night seeing is not as important as comfort in the daytime for preventing accidents.

Until 1969, tinted windshields were a separate option from tint in the remaining window glass. In this year the Chevrolet Division of General Motors began supplying all or no windows tinted. Tinted windshields alone are not available. This policy made it easier for the manufacturer to defend his logic that heat-absorbing windshields contribute to the comfort and hence to the safety of motoring. The heat argument is transparent when one notes the extra cost of this feature and the fact that the majority of cars on the highway, and virtually all of those produced by General Motors, have no heat insulation overhead. Thus, it appears that tinted windshields are a sales gimmick not greatly different from white sidewall tires and deluxe hubcaps.

THE AUTOMOBILE HORN

The horn is a great device for awakening people who may be day-dreaming at a traffic light. It has other "uses," such as calling the waitress at a drive-in, letting one's girl friend know he is driving by, and express-ing annoyance with another motorist. For safety its use is limited to those few occasions when—out of control, with wheels locked and tires skidding—a driver wants to tell a pedestrian, dog, or motorist to get braced or to run. The horn is usually listed as a safety device as, for ex-ample, in vehicle inspection laws. It probably was a safety device fifty years ago when vehicles traveled less than 30 mile per hour! If one pon-ders the placement of the horn in many vehicles, he finds that the sound is trapped in the engine compartment, where it is best heard by the driver himself. Few horn installations have the sound opening directed ahead, and few are free of obstructions to the direct emission of sound to the outside air!

Safety experts advise us to use our horn when we see someone en-croaching into our lane of travel on the highway. A simple analysis shows that this merely gives us something to do while we await the crash! Sound travels at 1,100 feet per second in calm air. Its intensity falls as the inverse square of the distance it travels. Thus if the sound has to travel 600 feet, its intensity will be about $\frac{1}{360,000}$ of its intensity at one foot from the horn. If the oncoming car has its windows closed, the sound must penetrate the glass, metal, and rubber of the automobile, with a fur-ther loss of its intensity. Even if the windows were open, the wind noises would mask the weakened horn sound.

Rarely mentioned in any safety literature is the use of headlights in-stead of the horn for highway communication. With light there is no loss of time in transmission, and the location of the signaling vehicle is in-stantly established. The brightness of the headlight is not reduced, even up to 1,700 feet away, at which distance its angular size becomes about 1 minute of arc. Beyond 1,700 feet the inverse square law holds; i.e., at 3,-400 feet the perceived brightness will be one fourth of what it was at 1,-700 feet. The probability of seeing a headlight in the highway situation just described is much better than hearing the horn. Effective visual warning can be given from distances well over 0.4 mile in good weather, or forty-two seconds in advance of the meeting point.

Safety literature, laws, and driver education courses should include the procedure of flashing headlights off and on, or from low to high, in rapid succession when it is necessary to warn oncoming traffic of your presence or of other hazards. The flashing of headlights with the horn button has been suggested by one inventor.

WATCHING FOR TURN OF FRONT WHEELS

Another favorite instruction by safety experts is to watch the front wheel of the oncoming car to detect when it first turns out of line. When a car is sitting at the curb, a turning of the steering wheel causes the front wheels to show the direction of travel before movement starts. As the car begins to move the effect of turning the wheel is more and more pronounced, so that at high speeds only a very slight movement of the steering wheel is required to move the car quickly from one side of the road to the other. In other words, the 1- or 2-degree movement of the front wheels would never be noticeable, although the displacement of the entire vehicle caused by it would. Only for very slow city driving can one rely on watching front wheels.

On the highway one has many more things to watch. Thus, gross displacements of vehicles are much easier to detect and are more reliable indices of hazard than front wheel aim. In fact, one should not and cannot depend upon central vision for anything in driving except studying those details brought to one's attention by peripheral vision. A search procedure of the entire scene is helpful, but without peripheral vision the totality and interrelationships of the perception could not be maintained. In short, attention should be paid to the car and its position on the pavement, to its speed and direction with respect to the whole scene, and to whether its general behavior foretells some unusual maneuver.

CENTRAL VS. PERIPHERAL ACUITY

The only test universally required by those states having driving licensing vision tests is central acuity. Peripheral acuity is not usually tested. Burg (1968) has shown that peripheral acuity does correlate, though weakly, with driving performance. Its importance in driving cannot be denied because it allows the inspection and interrelating of all the important objects in the field of view and allows the safe movement of the vehicle along the road, but to test central vision alone may pass a person with dangerous restrictions in his visual fields. A person with peripheral field problems may also be systemically sick and unfit to drive. A person with less than 180 degrees of horizontal visual field is abnormal.

Reductions of field from 180 to 140 degrees begins to be hazardous.

Similarly 20/40 vision is not enough for the safe operation of a motor vehicle at high speeds. For night driving, daytime 20/40 vision may become as poor as 20/200, depending upon the contrast of the target and the illuminance available. When we are being perceptually loaded more and more by increasing speeds and greater traffic density, we cannot afford to accept a daytime acuity to 20/40 when 20/20 or better is possible. The ultimate goal is the achievement of maximum visual performance for all drivers. Perhaps the way to accomplish this is to allow 20/20 or 20/25 as passing, with 20/30 and 20/40 as passing with warning and restriction to daytime driving. An acuity of 20/50 or worse should not pass. A review committee composed of optometrists, physicians, and Department of Motor Vehicle personnel should be called upon to study all aspects of an unsuccessful applicant's condition and situation if he is dissatisfied with the results of the vision and other tests he received.

YOUNG DRIVERS

By and large young drivers are inexperienced drivers. After World War II many Germans, thirty years of age and older, began to drive for the first time. Their accident experience curve looked much like that of the young drivers in the United States. The combination of inexperience on the highway and inexperience with alcohol accounts for part of young drivers' problems. Also, most young drivers drive more miles than older drivers, and the strongest correlation with driver accidents is the number of miles driven. The problem facing the young driver that is most often ignored is his old equipment. After you and I have used the safe miles in our cars, we despair of fixing all those little things like the worn brakes, worn tires, scratched windshield, misaligned front end, and worn shock absorbers, and we trade it in. Then, or after another owner or two, the kids get what's left over. Eager to prove they can drive like a pro, they push equipment to its limit. They learn what it can and cannot do, but some lose their lives or suffer heartbreaking injury when a critical part like a brake line, a tie rod end, a tire, a drive shaft, or a wheel bearing fails. Many survive because of skillful handling in the emergency and because of quick reactions.

The policy of insurance companies of dumping extra premium loads onto young nonvocal drivers is an added injustice to our potentially most useful citizens. It is also an indication of the indifference and selfishness of the adult population for allowing this to happen. In one college town police will stop a car full of college students for a minor infringement and often ignore townspeople who are doing the same thing. Upon identifying a driver as a member of the faculty and not a student, arresting officers have been known to fold up their ticket books, issuing only a verbal warning. Such discrimination against our youth is indeed unfair and unsettling.

Drivers above the age of about forty-five show a steady increase in accident rate. These, too, are often a deprived citizenry, driving an older family car or other automobile that gets serviced and cleaned less often than it should. After retirement, money and new cars do not come easily. The pace of the highway and city driving is increasing faster than they are prepared for, their reaction time is longer, their vision, hearing, and strength are impaired, and they are easily confused. That they have as few accidents as they do is a result of their small number compared to the larger numbers now driving at younger and younger ages. Their accident rate is held down somewhat by their increased experience and extra caution; nevertheless it is still almost as high as that of newly licensed drivers during their first three years.

To be fair, we should discriminate against our already disadvantaged older people as we do our youngsters, by raising their insurance rates too! It seems unreasonable and unfair to discriminate against any group based on age alone. However discrimination by higher insurance fees because of demonstrated inability to keep out of trouble, based on the number of violations and accidents compared to the number of miles driven, might have some preventive value.

LOOKING AT ONCOMING HEADLIGHTS

For the most part of the admonition to avoid looking at oncoming headlights for fear of being blinded for x number of seconds is of no practical importance and may in fact be hazardous! Suppose a long line of cars approaches with lights dimmed, as is most usually the case. Their lights, and your own, light the highway reasonably well, better than your lights alone would do. Now suppose there is a drunk driver behaving erratically in that line. If one watches only the right edge of the pavement, he may never see the collision developing, but if he watches the oncoming cars, he will be able to pick out those few cars that might cause trouble. In those states with paint stripes on the edge of the pavement, and with modern sealed-beam headlights, one can easily drive by peripheral vision while studying the oncoming headlights.

As to being blinded by such headlights, one can only blind the area where the bright image forms on the retina; all other areas are reasonably protected from the high intensities of direct headlight beams. Such localized bleaching of photopigment does not impair the ability to remain oriented by peripheral vision, since 98 percent of the rest of the retina is not bleached. Of some concern is the dirt on the outside of the windshield (which is no longer excusable since all new vehicles have windshield washers) and the hygroscopic smoke deposits on the inside of the windshield. When a bright headlight beam strikes such a windshield, it lights up all over and provides a significant bleaching effect over the entire retina which may require a few seconds for recovery. This is not an ocular deficiency but a windshield problem, and the solution is simple and obvious.

To watch oncoming automobiles tends to ignore pedestrians. However, pedestrians are not often encountered on open highways, and when they are they are usually not seen, whether one looks for them or not. Experiments show, as do accident statistics, that the chance of seeing a pedestrian in time to stop falls off markedly as speeds increase above 20 miles per hour. By 60 miles per hour, when driving with low headlights, as when meeting traffic, one might as well stop looking for pedestrians. If they are in the roadway it must be up to them to protect themselves. Reflectorized clothing, white or light colors, and significantly increased headlight power will solve this problem someday.

HIGH BEAM GLARE

In 1967 the Truckers of America felt the most hazardous thing a motorist could do at night was to drive with high beams. This point of view must have been reached from hearsay, because truck drivers as a rule sit so high that automobile high-beam headlights can scarcely interfere with their ability to see. In a series of driving tests made on interstate highways it was the truck driver in the lane over 100 feet to the side who most often asked that lights be dimmed, even though only about 3 percent of all drivers felt bothered enough to signal to dim. Rarely does one see truckers driving with high-beam headlights on, even on interstate highways. It has apparently not occurred to truck drivers, legislators, or anyone aside from a few researchers that the combination of 70 miles per hour (103 feet per second), a 300-foot maximum headlight range, a 2.5-second reaction time, and a stopping distance, once brakes are applied, of over 300 feet is not safe. Oblivious of the facts, everyone is fearful of blinding with high beams. Even the high-beam indicator light on most dash panels has a red warning light to signify danger!

On wide-open straight stretches of highway, one can see that high beams are safer than low. If two automobiles approach a mile or more apart with high beams, the roadway and shoulders between the two cars will be revealed. Soon, according to present law, the two drivers dim their lights. Suddenly areas of the road ahead are cloaked in darkness and visibility is worse. Now, unless obstacles, such as pedestrians, carry a light or retroreflective material, or unless the automobiles are equipped with special lighting, obstacles entering the pavement between the two cars will not be seen in time.

The Indiana Department of Motor Vehicles, as in most other states, admonishes all drivers to dim their headlights on interstate highways when meeting another car. That such dimming does not improve vision but impairs it and does not improve safety but causes a serious and obvious hazard must somehow be made clear to the nation. On divided highways high beams should not be optional but mandatory. The word of the trucker who literally sits above it all cannot be taken as the guideline for traffic safety when the facts are that low beams are inadequate even for 40 miles per hour. Even when overtaking, high beams should be permitted, since all new cars have inside mirrors that can be tilted to reduce their brightness. Less distress would occur to the passed driver if he were also driving with high beams as here recommended. If the all-weather headlighting system recommended in Chapter 8 were adopted, there would be practically no problems with glare, either from the front or rear, since the eye level zone of headlighting would be free of light.

Bibliography

Abbott Laboratories. "Glaucoma," *What's New* (North Chicago, Ill.), 1962.

ABELSON, PHILIP H. "A Damaging Source of Air Pollution," *Science,* Vol. 158, No. 3808, Dec. 22, 1967.

ABERNETHY, ROY. "We Care Very Much," *Highway User,* Vol. 30, No. 5, May 1965, 16–17.

"Accident Prevention Spotlighted at Annual SAE Meeting," *Traffic Safety,* March 1968, 16–18ff.

ADAMS, ANTHONY J., and JOHN R. LEVENE. "Stereoscopic Depth Associated with Cyclotorsional Eye Movements," *British Journal of Physiological Optics,* Vol. 24, No. 3, 1967, 217–220.

ADAMS, JAMES R., and E. BELVIN WILLIAMS. "Association Between Smoking and Accidents; Overdependency as an Influencing Variable," *Traffic Quarterly,* Vol. 20, No. 4, Oct. 1966, 583–588.

ADAMS, LEON D. "Stupid Highway Signs Can Kill," *Popular Science,* Vol. 186, No. 5, May 1965, 104–108ff.

ADLER, F. H. *Physiology of the Eye,* C. V. Mosby Co., St. Louis, Mo., 1965.

ADRIAN, WERNER. "Principles of Disability and Discomfort Glare," *Proceedings, Symposium on Visibility in the Driving Task,* sponsored by Highway Research Board, Illuminating Engineering Research Institute, and Texas A & M University, May 13–15, 1968, 75–95.

ADY, R. W. "Investigation of the Relationship between Illuminated Advertising Signs and Expressway Accidents," *Traffic Safety Research Review,* Vol. 11, No. 1, 1967, 9–11.

Aerospace Systems Safety Society. *Hazard Prevention,* Vol. 3, No. 3, Dec. 1965.

"Alcohol and Vision Experiment," *Accident Facts, 1967* (New York State Department of Motor Vehicles), 15.

"Alcohol in Perspective," *Consumer Reports,* Vol. 31, No. 2, Feb. 1967, 97–99.

"Alcohol or CO Found in Half the Driver Dead," *Highway Research Abstracts,* Vol. 36, No. 6, June 1966, 3.

ALLEN, MERRILL J. "Influence of Age on the Speed of Accommodation," *American Journal of Optometry and Archives of American Academy of Optometry,* Vol. 199, 1956.

———. *Study of Visual Performance Using Ophthalmic Filters,* A.S.D. Technical Report 61-576, Wright Patterson Air Force Base, Ohio, Oct. 1961, 29 pp.

———. "How Do You Fit Spectacles?" *Indiana Journal of Optometry,* Vol. 32, No. 2, April 1962, 5–7.

———. "Effective Means of Increasing Highway Illumination and Reducing the Headlight Glare," *Journal of the American Optometric Association,* Vol. 34, No. 3, Oct. 1962, 225–226.

———. "Indiana State Fair Vision Screening Booth," *Indiana Journal of Optometry,* Vol. 32, No. 4, Oct. 1962, 10–11.

———. "Certain Visual Aspects of the Average Modern American Automobile," *Journal of the American Optometric Association,* Vol. 34, No, 5, Dec. 1962, 380–383.

————. "On Automobile Auxiliary Side Lights," *Science News Letter*, Jan. 26, 1963.

————. "Daytime Automobile Windshield and Dash Panel Characteristics," *American Journal of Optometry and Archives of American Academy of Optometry*, Vol. 40, No. 2, Feb. 1963, 61–72.

————. "Special Motor Vehicle Auxiliary Lights Designed to Reduce the Effects of Glare and Aid Highway Visibility," *Highway Research News*, No. 5, May 1963, 24.

————. "Glasses for Automobile Driving?" *Optometric Weekly*, Vol. 54, No. 48, Nov. 28, 1963, 2238–2239.

————. "Volkswagen's 'Outlook,'" *Small World* (VW of America, Englewood Cliffs, N. J.), Vol. 2, No. 4, Fall 1963.

————. "Automobile Running Lights, A Research Report," *American Journal of Optometry and Archives of American Academy of Optometry*, Vol. 41, No. 5, May 1964, 293–315.

————. "Eye Injuries in Automobile Accidents," *Journal of the American Optometric Association*, Vol. 35, No. 7, July 1964, 623.

————. "Automobiles and Yellow Lights," *Journal of the American Optometric Association*, Vol. 35, No. 7, July 1964, 607.

————. "Painted Bulbs in Turn Signals Dangerous," *Journal of the American Optometric Association*, Vol. 35, No. 6, Aug. 1964, 662.

————. "Automobiles and Yellow Lights, Part II," *Journal of the American Optometric Association*, Vol. 35, No. 10, Oct. 1964, 871–872.

————. "Automobile Dash Panel Visibility Impairment Due to Wearing Fit-Over Sunglasses," *American Journal of Optometry and Archives of American Academy of Optometry*, Vol. 41, No. 10, Oct. 1964, 595–598.

————. "Vision Screening at Indiana State Fair," *Journal of the American Optometric Association*, Vol. 35, No. 11, Nov. 1964, 974–977.

————. "Misuse of Red Light on Automobiles," *American Journal of Optometry and Archives of American Academy of Optometry*, Vol. 41, No. 12, Dec. 1964, 695–699.

————. "Running Light Questionnaire," *American Journal of Optometry and Archives of American Academy of Optometry*, Vol. 42, No. 3, March 1965, 164–167.

————. "Visibility Problems Cause Automobile Accidents," *Indiana University Review*, Vol. 7, No. 3, May 1, 1965, 1–6.

————. "Tinted Windshields Are a Hazard!" *Optometric Weekly*, May 6, 1965, 76–77.

————. "Automobile Visibility Problems," *Journal of the American Optometric Association*, Vol. 36, No. 9, Sept. 1965, 807–810.

————. "Eye Position on the Highway," *Journal of the American Optometric Association*, Vol. 37, No. 5, May 1966, 460.

————. "Automobile Windshields, A New Car Study, 1966 Models," *Optometric Weekly*, Vol. 57, No. 28, July 14, 1966, 14–17.

————. "Vision, Vehicles, and Highway Safety," *Highway Research News*, No. 25, Autumn 1966, 57–62.

————. "How to Avoid Dying with Your Boots On," *Bulletin of the Woman's Auxiliary to the American Optometric Association*, Vol. 21, No. 2, Nov. 1966, 6.

————. "Chromium Headlight Covers, A Possible Hazard," *American Journal of Optometry and Archives of American Academy of Optometry*, Vol. 44, No. 1, Jan. 1967, 34–41.

————. "Visual Environment in the Modern Automobile," Prevention of Highway Injury Symposium, University of Michigan Highway Safety Research Institute, April 1967, 118–121.

————. "Tips for the Older Driver," *Optometric Weekly*, Vol. 58, No. 23, June 8, 1967, 31–32.

————. "Headlight Ring Retro-reflectors," *American Journal of Optometry and Archives of American Academy of Optometry*, Vol. 44, No. 12, Dec. 1967, 765–768.

————. "Report on Windshield Tint and Angles," *Physicians for Automobile Safety News Letter* (537 Morris Ave., Springfield, N.J.), April, 1968.

————. "Glare and Driver Vision Report," Contract FH-11-6550, National Highway Safety Bureau, submitted Spring 1968.

————. "Disappearing Headlights," *Journal of the American Optometric Association,* Vol. 40, No. 6, June 1969, 601–602.

————. "Automobile Windshields—Surface Deterioration," *American Journal of Optometry and Archives of American Academy of Optometry,* Aug. 1969, 594–958.

————. "Chrysler Corporation's Super-Lite, An Evaluation," *American Journal of Optometry and Archives of American Academy of Optometry,* Nov. 1969.

————, and WILLIAM M. LYLE. "Relationship Between Night Driving Ability and the Amount of Light Needed for a Specific Performance on a Low Contrast Target," *Journal of the American Optometric Association,* Vol. 34, No. 16, Nov. 1963, 1301–1303.

————, and JOHN H. CARTER. "Visual Problems Associated with Motor Vehicle Driving at Dusk," *Journal of the American Optometric Association,* Vol. 35, No. 1, Jan. 1964.

————, and JOHN K. CROSLEY. "Automobile Liquid Glass Tint, A Research Report," *American Journal of Optometry and Archives of American Academy of Optometry,* Vol. 42, No. 6, June 1965, 344–350.

————, and ————. "Automobile Liquid Glass Tint," *Highway Research Abstracts,* Vol. 36, No. 3, March 1966, 6.

————, and ————. "Auxiliary Lighting to Improve Rear Visibility of Trucks and Buses," *American Journal of Optometry and Archives of American Academy of Optometry,* Vol. 44, No. 5, May 1967.

————, and G.R. COURTNEY. "Photomyoclonic and Photoconvulsive Responses to Flickering Light," *Journal of the American Optometric Association,* Vol. 38, No. 2, Feb. 1967, 111–112.

————, JERALD STRICKLAND, and ANTHONY J. ADAMS. "Visibility of Red, Green, Amber, and White Signal Lights in a Highway Scene," *American Journal of Optometry and Archives of American Academy of Optometry,* Vol. 44, No. 2, Feb. 1967, 105–109.

————, and JOHANNES J. VOS. "Ocular Scattered Light and Visual Performance as a Function of Age," *American Journal of Optometry and Archives of American Academy of Optometry,* Vol. 44, No. 11, Nov. 1967, 717–727.

————, *et al.* "Visibility Distances of a Pedestrian, With and Without Glare, and the Pedestrian's Estimation of His Own Visibility," *American Journal of Optometry and Archives of American Academy of Optometry,* Dec. 1969.

ALLEN, T. M. "Visibility of Signs," *Proceedings, Symposium on Visibility in the Driving Task,* sponsored by Highway Research Board, Illuminating Engineering Research Institute, and Texas A & M University, May 13–15, 1968, paper not avail.

————, and A. L. STRAUB. "Sign Brightness and Legibility," *Highway Research Board Bulletin* 127, 1955, 1–14.

ALLGAIER, E. "Better Visibility for Civilian Night Driving," *Optometric Weekly,* Vol. 51, 1960, 2570–2573.

————. "Better Vision Makes Better Drivers," *Journal of the American Optometric Association,* Vol. 32, 1960, 217–219.

ALPERN, S. E. "Contact Lenses and Automobile Driving," *Journal of the American Optometric Association,* Vol. 32, 1960, 221–223.

American Association for Automotive Medicine. *Pre-Crash Factors in Traffic Safety,* 12th Annual Symposium, Sacramento, Calif., 1968.

American Automobile Association. *Seat Belts for Passenger Cars* (1712 G Street NW, Washington, D.C.), 1963.

————. *Foundation for Traffic Safety: Manual on Pedestrian Safety* (Washington, D.C.), 1964.

————. *Driver Education Equipment* (Washington, D.C.), 1965.

"American Massacre," *American Trial Lawyers, I,* No. 1, Dec. 1964.

American Optometric Association. *Manual on Drivers' Vision Test,* St. Louis, Mo., 1949.

American Trial Lawyers Association. *Stop Murder by Motor,* New York, 1966.

ANDREOTTI, FRANCESCO. "Universal Type of Metal Number Plate in All Countries of the World," *International Police Chronicle,* No. 70, Jan.–Feb. 1965, 45–51.

"Antiskid Road Works," *Science News,* Vol. 95, Jan. 4, 1969, 14.

"Are You a Defensive Driver?" *U.S. Navy Medical News Letter*, Vol. 48, No. 7, Oct. 1966, 22.

ARMAND, HARRY. "Make the Automobile Safer," *Safety Engineering*, parts 1–15, Jan. 1937 to March 1938.

———. "Criticism and Safer Automobiles," *Safety Engineering*, Feb. 1938.

———. "This Year It's Hudson," *Safety Engineering*, Nov. 1940, 14–16, 34.

ARMISTEAD, W. H., and S. D. STOOKEY. "Photochromic Silicate Glasses Sensitized by Silver Halides," *Science*, Vol. 144, April 1964, 150–154.

ATKIN, DOROTHY. "Safety Forum: Running Lights in Daytime?" *Fleet Owner*, Jan. 1965, 138–139.

"Atmospheric Opacity, a Study of Visibility Observations in the British Isles," *Quarterly Journal of Royal Meteorological Society*, Vol. 65, 411–442, 1939.

Automotive Safety Foundation. "Railroad Grade Crossings," *Traffic Control Elements: Their Relationship to Highway Safety/Revised*, Chapter I, Washington, D.C., 1968.

———. "Traffic Volume," *Traffic Control Elements: Their Relationship to Highway Safety/Revised*, Chapter II, Washington, D.C., 1969.

———. "Illumination," *Traffic Control and Roadway Elements: Their Relationship to Highway Safety/Revised*, Chapter III, Washington, D.C., 1969.

AULHORN, E. "Die Blendung aus der Sicht des Ophthalmologen," *Berichte dei Deutschen Ophthalmologischen Gesellschaftin Heidelberg*, Vol. 65, 1963, 454.

———. "Uber die Beziehung zwischen Lichtsinn und Sehscharfe," *Albrecht von Graefe's Archiv fur Ophthalmologie*, Vol. 4, 1964, 167.

———. and H. HARMS. "Untersuchungen uber das Wesen des Grenzkontrastes," *Berichte der Deutschen Ophthalmologischen Gesellschaft in Heidelberg*, Vol. 60, 1956, 7.

Automobile Manufacturers Association. *The State of the Art of Traffic Safety*, Part 1, Arthur D. Little, Cambridge, Mass., 1966, 16–31.

———. *1968/Automobile Facts/Figures*, Detroit, Mich., 1968.

Automotive Medicine Association. "Effect of Drugs on Drivers' Vision Stressed," *Medical Tribune and Medical News*, Vol. 8, No. 119, Dec. 11, 1967, 24.

"Automotive Safety and Engineering Responsibility," *American Engineer*, Oct. 1965, 31–36.

Automotive Safety Research Office. *Data on the Motor Vehicle Transportation System in the United States, A Delineation of the Motor Vehicle Accident Problem*, Engineering Staff, Ford Motor Company (Dearborn, Mich., 48121), Nov. 1968.

"Auxiliary Lights Urged," *Automotive Industries*, Feb. 1, 1963, 26.

BAGLIEN, J. W. "Driving Vision," *Optometric Weekly*, Vol. 51, 1960, 1811–1814.

BAILEY, NEAL J., and HENRY W. HOFSTETTER. "Effect of Ophthalmic Lens Fluorescence on Visual Acuity," *American Journal of Optometry and Archives of American Academy of Optometry*, Vol. 36, 1959, 634.

BAKER, C. A., and W. C. STEEDMAN. "Perceived Movement in Depth as a Function of Luminance and Velocity," *Human Factors*, Vol. 3, No. 3, 1961, 166.

BALL, R. J., and S. HOWARD BARTLEY. "Induction and Reduction of Color Deficiency by Manipulation of Temporal Aspects of Photic Input," *American Journal of Optometry and Archives of American Academy of Optometry*, Vol. 44, No. 7, July 1967, 411–418.

BALUYUT, LOLITA C., and HENRY W. HOFSTETTER. "Statistical Review of 1,000 Vision Certificates," *Journal of the American Optometric Association*, Vol. 35, No. 8, August 1964, 664–668.

BANKS, ANDERSON. "Retinal Responses to Ischemia and Hyperoxia," *North Carolina Medical Journal*, Vol. 26, Oct. 1965, 446–449.

BARACH, A. L., ROSS A. McFARLAND, and C. P. SEITZ. "Effects of Oxygen Deprivation on Complex Medical Functions," *Journal of Aviation Medicine*, Vol. 8, No. 4, 1937, 197–207.

BARBARIK, PAUL. "Auto Accidents and Driver Reaction Patterns," *Journal of Applied Psychology*, Vol. 52, No. 1, 1968, 49–54.

BARMACK, J. E., *et al.* "Field Evaluation of the Smith-Cummings-Sherman Driver Performance Rating Scale," *Traffic Safety Research Review,* Vol. 6, No. 2, 1962, 25–30.

——, and D. E. PAYNE. "Injury-producing Private Motor Vehicle Accidents Among Airmen: Psychological Models of Accident Generating Process," *Traffic Safety Research Review,* Vol. 6, No. 3, 1962, 24–32.

BARTLETT, N. R., and S. MacLEOD. "Effect of Flash and Field Luminance Upon Human Reaction Time," *Journal of the Optical Society of America,* Vol. 44, No. 4, 1954, 306–311.

BARTLEY, S. HOWARD. "What Optometrists Should Know About Fatigue," *Michigan Optometrist,* March 1952.

——. G. PACZEWITZ, and E. VALSI. "Brightness Enhancement and the Stimulus Cycle," *Journal of Psychology,* Vol. 43, 1957, 187.

BELZER, E. G., and W. J. HUFFMAN. "Quickness of Selected Right-foot and Left-foot Braking Techniques," *Traffic Safety Research Review,* Vol. 10, No. 3, 1966, 72–77.

BERGER, C. *et al.* "Effect of Anoxia on Visual Resolving Power," *American Journal of Psychology,* Vol. 56, July 1943, 395–407.

BERGEVIN, J., and MICHAEL MILLODOT. "Glare with Ophthalmic and Corneal Lenses," *American Journal of Optometry and Archives of American Academy of Optometry,* Vol. 44, April 1967, 213–221.

BEWLEY, LAWRENCE A. "Spectacle Frames Reduce the Field of Vision: A Driving Hazard," *Journal of the American Optometric Association,* Vol. 40, No. 1, Jan. 1969, 64–69.

BHATIA, B. "Some Factors Determining the Maximum Angular Velocity of Pursuit Ocular Movements," *Journal of the Optical Society of America,* Vol. 50, 1960, 149–150.

BICKFORD, R. G. "Thresholds for Production of Seizures by Photic Stimulation in Man," *American Journal of Physiology,* Vol. 155, 1948, 427 (abstract).

BIRKHOFF, A. J., and H. R. BLACKWELL. "A Visual Evaluation of Illumination in the Roadway Environment," Proj. HR63–5–2 *National Cooperative Highway Research Program, Institute for Research in Vision and Transport,* Sept. 1966, 1–42.

BIRREN, FABER. "Safety on the Highway: A Problem of Vision, Visibility, and Color," *American Journal of Ophthalmology,* Vol. 43, No. 2, 1957, 265–270.

BLACKWELL, H. R. "Effect of Tinted Optical Media upon Visual Efficiency at Low Luminance," *Journal of the Optical Society of America,* Vol. 43, 1953, 815.

——. "Visual Detection at Low Luminance through Optical Filters," *Highway Research Board Bulletin 89,* 1954, 43.

——. "Use of Visual Brightness Discrimination Data in Illuminating Engineering," Commission Internationale de l'Eclairage, 13th Session, Zurich, 1955.

——. "Visual Capabilities of the Automobile Driver," Report of the Armed Forces-National Research Council Committee on Vision Symposium on the Visual Factors in Automobile Driving, *National Academy of Sciences—National Research Council Publication 574,* Washington, D.C., 1958, 8–9.

——. "Discussion of Paper Entitled 'Practical Application of Polarization and Light Control for Reduction of Reflected Glare,'" by C. L. Crouch and J. E. Kaufman, *Illuminating Engineering,* Vol. 58, 1963, 283–290.

——. "Visibility of Signals," *Proceedings, Symposium on Visibility in the Driving Task,* sponsored by Highway Research Board, Illuminating Engineering Research Institute, and Texas A & M University, May 13–15, 1968, 146–154.

——. and O. M. BLACKWELL, "Visibility of Objects on Highways," *Proceedings, Symposium on Visibility in the Driving Task,* sponsored by Highway Research Board, Illuminating Engineering Research Institute, and Texas A & M University, May 13–15, 1968, 106–123.

——, and B. S. PRITCHARD. "New Instruments for Field Measurements of Illumination Requirements and Disability Glare," *Proceedings, 3rd Research Symposium of the Illuminating Engineering Research Institute,* New York, 1961, 10.

————, and ————. "Sight Through Fog," *Proceedings, 3rd Research Symposium of the Illuminating Engineering Research Institute,* New York, 1961, 10.

————, ————, and R. N. SCHWAB. "Illumination Requirements for Roadway Visual Tasks," *Highway Research Board Bulletin 255,* 1960, 117–127.

————, ————, and ————. "Light for Safety on Streets and Roadways," *Proceedings, 3rd Research Symposium of the Illuminating Engineering Research Institute,* New York, 1961, 16.

————, ————, and ————. *Test Data on Visibility and Illumination Variables in Roadway Visual Tasks,* Ohio State University, Institute for Research in Vision and Engineering Experiment Station, Report on Project 47, Illuminating Engineering Research Institute, 1963, 50.

————, ————, and ————. "Visibility and Illumination Variables in Roadway Visual Tasks," *Illuminating Engineering,* Vol. 59, No. 5, Sec. I, May 1964, 277.

————, ————, and ————. "Illumination Variables in Visual Tasks of Drivers," *Public Roads,* Vol. 33, No. 11, 1965, 237–248.

BLANCHE, ERNEST E. "Roadside Distraction," *Traffic Safety,* Vol. 65, No. 11, Nov. 1965, 24–25, 36–37.

BLIKRA, GEORG, and ROLF RINGKJØB. "Personskader Ved Trafikkulykker, Behandlet I Ulleval Sykehus 1966" (Personal Injuries Caused by Traffic Accidents, Treated at Ulleval Hospital, 1966), *Report No. 2, UTVALG for Trafikksikker-Netsforskning,* Statsjousveien 4, Oslo, Sentralboro 608280, Slemdal, Aug. 1968.

BOELTER and RYDER. "Notes on the Behavior of a Beam of Light in Fog," *Illuminating Engineering,* Vol. 35, 1940.

BOETTNER, A. E., and J. R. WOLTER. *Transmission of the Ocular Media,* Technical Documentary Report No. MRL-TDR-62-34, Wright-Patterson Air Force Base, Ohio, May 1962. Also in *Investigative Ophthalmology,* Vol. 1, No. 6, Dec. 1962, 776–783.

BOX, PAUL C. "Driver Age as Related to Freeway Accidents," *Proceedings, Symposium on Visibility in the Driving Task,* sponsored by Highway Research Board, Illuminating Engineering Research Institute, and Texas A & M University, May 13–15, 1968, 44–55.

BOYNTON, ROBERT M., and FRANK J. CLARKE. "Sources of Entoptic Scatter in the Human Eye," *Journal of the Optical Society of America,* Vol. 54, No. 1, Jan. 1964, 110–119.

BRECHER, GERHARD A., A. P. HARTMAN, and D. D. LEONARD. "Effect of Alcohol on Binocular Vision," *American Journal of Ophthalmology,* Vol. 39, No. 2, pt. 2, 1955, 44–52.

BRECKENRIDGE, F. C. *United States Standard for the Colors of Signal Lights,* U. S. Department of Commerce, Washington, D. C., 1964.

BRODY, L. "Role of Vision in Motor Vehicle Operation," *International Record of Medicine,* Vol. 167, June 1954, 365–377.

BOMBRACH, T. A. "Contact Lenses and Visual Fields," *Contacto,* Aug. 1961, 265–277.

BROSCHMANN, D. "To the Question of Driving Ability in Uniocular Mydriasis," *Klinische Monatsblätter für Augenheilkunde,* 1967, 151, 116–119.

BROWN, EDWARD G. *Report of Reflectorization of License Plates,* Joint Committee on Highways, Washington State Legislature, 1964, 1–3.

BROWN, R. H. "Analysis of Visual Sensitivity to Differences in Velocity," *U.S. Naval Research Laboratory Report 5478,* 1960, 16 pp.

————. "Weber Ratio for Visual Discrimination of Velocity," *Science,* Vol. 131, 1960, 1809–1810.

BRYAN, W. E. "Research in Vision and Traffic Safety," *Journal of the Optometric Association,* Vol. 29, No. 3, Oct. 1957, 169–172.

————. "Lenses for Night Driving," *Highway Research Board Bulletin 336,* Jan. 1962, 104.

————, and HENRY W. HOFSTETTER. "Statistical Summary and Evaluation of the Vision of Automobile Drivers," *Journal of the American Optometric Association,* Vol. 29, 1958, 513.

BUGELSKI, B. R. "Traffic Signals and Depth Perception," *Science,* Vol. 157, 1967, 1464.

Bureau of Public Roads. *Federal Role in Highway Safety* (A Report to Congress), 1959.

BURG, ALBERT. "Visual Acuity as Measured by Dynamic and Static Tests: A Comparative Evaluation," *Journal of Applied Psychology*, Vol. 50, No. 6, 1966, 460–466.

————. "Relationship Between Vision Test Scores and Driving Record: General Findings," University of California Department of Engineering, 1967.

————. "Horizontal Phoria as Related to Age and Sex," *American Journal of Optometry and Archives of American Academy of Optometry*, Vol. 45, No. 6, June 1968, 345–350.

————. "Relation Between Vison Quality and Driving Record," *Proceedings, Symposium on Visibility in the Driving Task*, sponsored by Highway Research Board, Illuminating Engineering Research Institute, and Texas A & M University, May 13–15, 1968, 5–16.

————. *Vision Test Scores and Driving Record: Additional Findings*, Institute of Transportation and Traffic Engineering, California Department of Motor Vehicles, Dec. 1968.

————, and S. F. HULBERT. "Dynamic Visual Acuity and Other Measures of Vision," *Perception and Motor Skills*, Vol. 9, 1959, 334.

————, and ————. "Dynamic Visual Acuity as Related to Age, Sex, and Static Acuity," *Journal of Applied Psychology*, Vol. 45, No. 2, 1961, 111–116.

BYRNES, VISTOR A. "Visual Factors in Automobile Driving," *Transactions of the American Ophthalmological Society*, Vol. 60, 1962, 60–79.

————. "Vision and Its Importance in Driving," *Sight-Saving Review*, Vol. 37, No. 2, Summer 1967, 87–90.

CADLE, R. D. *Particle Size Determination*, Interscience Publishers, New York, 1955.

California Department of Motor Vehicles. *Vision Research Project Progress Report*, Research Report No. 2, Oct. 1, 1959.

California Highway Patrol. *Motorcycle Accident Study* (P. O. Box 898, Sacramento, Calif. 95804), Jan. 1968.

CAMPBELL, B. J., and W. S. ROUSE. "Reflectorized License Plates and Rear End Collisions at Night," *Traffic Safety Research Review*, Vol. 12, No. 2, June 1968, 40–45.

CAMPBELL, H. E. "Carbon Monoxide, Smoking in Automobiles and Haylofts," *Journal of the American Medical Association*, Vol. 207, No. 5, Feb. 3, 1969, 951.

"Canada Instituting Uniform Traffic Sign, Signal and Marking Program," *Highway Research News*, 42–43.

CHALFONT, M. W. "Who the Problem Drivers Are," *Optometric Weekly*, Vol. 52, 1961, 2311–2312.

CHAPMAN, ALBERT L. "Accident Prevention," *Pennsylvania Medical Journal*, Vol. 61, Sept. 1958, 1201–1203.

CHESEBROUGH, HARRY E. "Cars in the Future—An Engineer Dreams Ahead." *Highway Research Abstracts*, Vol. 36, No. 6, June 1966, 15.

CHESSMAN, MAX R., and WILLIAM T. VOSS. *Motor Vehicle Headlight Beam Usage Study on a Section of Interstate Highway 90 in South Dakota*, South Dakota Department of Highway Research and Planning Division, 1964.

CHRISTIE, A. W. "Night Accident Problem and the Effect of Public Lighting," Reprinted from the *Journal of the Association of Public Lighting Engineers, Public Lighting*, Vol. 33, No. 141, June 1968, 98–101.

————, and A. J. FISHER. "Effect of Glare from Street Lighting Lanterns on the Visibility of Objects for Drivers of Different Ages," *Proceedings of the Third Conference of the Australian Road Research Board*, Vol. 3, Part 1, 1966, 570–588.

CIBIS, PAUL A., and FRITZ HABER. *Studies on Effects of Windshields and/or Air of Different Densities on Stereoscopic Vision*, Mathematical Principles concerning Displacement Effects on Bidimensional Perception of Direction, Size, and Distance, and Tridimensional Perception of Depth, Unnumbered project report No. 1, Department of Ophthalmology, USAF School of Aviation Medicine (Randolph Field), Texas, Nov. 1950.

————, and MAX HALPERIN. *Faulty Depth Perception Caused by Cyclotorsion of the Eyes*, USAF School of Aviation Medicine Project Report, Texas, 1951.

COBB, PERCY W., and FRANK K. MOSS. "Four Variables of the Visual Threshold," *Journal of the Franklin Institute*, Vol. 205, No. 6, June 1928, 831–847.

————, and ————. "Effect of Dark Surroundings upon Vision," *Journal of the Franklin Institute*, Vol. 206, No. 6, Dec. 1928, 827–840.

COCKE *et al.* "Chloramphenicol Optic Toxicity," *Journal of Pediatrics*, Vol. 68, Jan. 1966, 27.

COLDWELL, B. B. "Highway Investigations (Effects of Alcohol)," *R.C.M.P. Quarterly* (Royal Canadian Mounted Police, Ottawa, Canada), Vol. 31, No. 2, Oct. 1965, 17–24.

COLE, BEN. "Blinking Devices May Cut Traffic Toll," *Indianapolis Star*, Sept. 19, 1965, 1.

COLE, B. L. "Distribution of Intensity for Road Traffic Light Signals," *Australian Road Research*, Vol. 2, 1966, 13–20.

————, *et al.* "Transport Lighting," *Australian Road Research*, Vol. 2, No. 6, Dec. 1965, 51–57.

————, and B. BROWN. "Intensity of In-Service Road Traffic Signal Lights," *Australian Road Research*, Vol. 2, No. 6, Dec. 1965, 58–69.

————, and ————. "Note on the Effectiveness of Surround Screens for Road Traffic Lights," *Australian Road Research*, Vol. 2, 1966, 21–23.

————, and ————. "Preliminary Examination of the Optical Performance of Road Traffic Signal Lights," *Australian Road Research*, Vol. 2, 1966, 24–32.

————, and ————. "Optimum Intensity of Red Road Traffic Signal Lights for Normal and Protanopic Observers," *Journal of the Optical Society of America*, Vol. 56, 1966, 516–522.

————, and ————. "Specification of Road Traffic Signal Light Intensity," *Human Factors*, Vol. 10, 1968, 245–254.

————, and ————, "Effect of Visual Noise on the Visibility of Road Traffic Signal Lights," *Australian Road Research*, in press.

————, discussion in B.A.J. Clark, "Effects of Tinted Ophthalmic Media on the Recognition of Red Traffic Signals," *Australian Road Research*, in press.

COLLINS, WILLIAM E. "Vestibular Responses from Figure Skaters," *Aerospace Medicine*, Office of Aviation Medicine, Civil Aeromedical Institute, Federal Aviation Agency (Oklahoma City, Okla. 73101), Nov. 1966, 1098–1104.

Colorado State Department of Highways. "Colorado's Reflective Bead Study," Planning and Research Division (4201 Arkansas Ave., Denver, Col. 80222), Nov. 1968.

"Colored Pavements," *Traffic Safety*, March 1968, 26.

COLSON, W. "Effect of Alcohol on Vision," *Journal of the American Medical Association*, Vol. 115, Nov. 2, 1940, 1525–1526.

CONNERS, M. M., and J. A. S. KINNEY. "Relative Red-Green Sensitivity as a Function of Retinal Position," *Journal of the Optical Society of America*, Vol. 52, 1962, 81–84.

CONNOLLY, PAUL L. "Vision and Headlight Glare," *Michigan Optometrist*, Vol. 16, No. 5, May 1947.

————. "Recent Developments in Automotive Lighting," Monograph 305, *American Journal of Optometry and Archives of American Academy of Optometry*, Aug. 1962, 415.

————. "In the Vehicle and On the Road," Society of Automotive Engineers publication SP-253, March 1964.

————. "About Cars and Vision," *Industrial Design*, Part I, Vol. 11, No. 1, Jan. 1964, 38; Part II, Vol. 12, No. 5, May 1965, 66.

————. "Automobiles, Vision and Driving," *Optometric Weekly*, Vol. 56, No. 48, Dec. 1965, 26–28; Vol. 57, No. 2, Jan. 1966, 36–38.

————. "Visual Considerations: Man, the Vehicle, and the Highway," *Police*, July-August, 1966.

————. "An Optometrist Analyzes Safe Driver Vision," *Autoproducts* (Cummins Publishing Co., Oak Park, Mich.), Vol. 4, No. 8, Aug. 1966.

———. "Vision, Man, Vehicle and Highway," reprinted from *Prevention of Highway Injury,* Proceedings from Symposium, University of Michigan Highway Safety Research Institute, 1967.

———. "Human and Visual Factors Considerations for the Design of Automotive Periscopic Systems," Society of Automotive Engineers Mid-Year Meeting, Detroit, May 20-24, 1968.

———, and INGEBORG SCHMIDT. *Visual Considerations of Man, the Vehicle and the Highway,* SP-279, 1966.

———, W. A. DEVLIN, JR., and KONRAD H. MARCUS. "Design Aspects for Rear Vision in Motor Vehicles," SP-253 presented at SAE Automobile Meeting, Detroit, March 1964.

———, ———, and ———. "A Look to the Rear with an Eye to Safety," *SAE Journal,* Vol. 73, No. 7, July 1965, 30–41.

COPPIN, R. S., *et al.* "Effectiveness of Short Individual Driver Improvement Sessions," *Highway Research Abstracts,* Vol. 36, No. 6, June 1966, 3.

Cornell Aeronautical Laboratory. "ACIR Evaluates Safety of New Windshield," *Transportation Research Review* (Buffalo, N.Y.), Third/Fourth Quarter 1968.

"Countdown Traffic Light Ticks off Seconds," *Popular Science,* June 1966, 131.

"Country Driving Dangers Outlined," *AMA News,* March 21, 1966, 3.

CRANCER, A., *et al.* "Comparison of the Effects of Marihuana and Alcohol on Simulated Driving Performance," *Science,* Vol. 164, No. 3881, May 16, 1969, 851–854.

CRANDELL, FRANK J. *Packaging the Passenger,* Liberty Mutual Insurance Company (Boston, Mass.).

CRAWFORD, W. A. "Perception of Moving Objects: II. Eye Movements," RAF Flying Personnel Research Commission, Farnborough, England. Memo 150b, July 1960.

CRESSWELL, W. L., and P. FROGGATT. "Causation of Bus Driver Accidents," published by Oxford University Press for Nuffield Provincial Hospitals Trust, London, 1963, 101–102.

CRINIGAN, R. P. "Survey of Motorists' Vision Requirements," *Traffic Safety Research Review,* Vol. 4, No. 3, 1960, 29–32, and *Journal of the American Optometric Association,* Vol. 32, 1960, 209–210.

CROSLEY, JOHN, and MERRILL J. ALLEN. "Automobile Brake Light Effectiveness: An Evaluation of High Placement and Accelerator Switching," *American Journal of Optometry and the Archives of the American Academy of Optometry,* Vol. 43, No. 5, May 1966, 299–304.

CROSS, MILLAR, and SIMPSON. "Vital Importance of Fixed Lighting on Public Roads," *Illuminating Engineering,* Vol. 41, 1946.

CUMMING, R. W. "Analysis of Skills in Driving," *Australian Road Research,* Vol. 1, No. 9, March 1964, 4–14.

DAMON, A., and Ross A. McFARLAND. "Physique of Bus and Truck Drivers: With a Review of Occupational Anthropology," *American Journal of Physical Anthropology,* Vol. 13, No. 4, Dec. 1955, 711–742.

DANIELSON, R. W. "Relationship of Fields of Vision to Safety in Driving," *American Journal of Ophthalmology,* Vol. 44, No. 5, Part I, Nov. 1957, 657–680.

DARRELL, J. E. P., and M. D. BUNNETTE. "Driver Performance Related to Interchange Marking and Nighttime Visibility Conditions," Highway Research Board Bulletin 137, 1960, 128–137.

DAVEY, J. B. "Road Safety: Some Visual Aspects," *Optician,* Vol. 139, 1960, 436–438.

———. "Vision and Eye Movements of Auto Drivers," *Optician,* Vol. 140, 1961, 676.

———. "Visual Task of Road Users," *Optician,* Vol. 141, 1962, 669–673.

———. "Reflections at the Motor Show," *Ophthalmic Optician,* Nov. 28, 1964, 1205–1214.

———. "Incidence and Causes of Blindness in England and Wales, 1948–1962," *Ophthalmic Optician,* April 2, 1966, 325–327.

———. "Night Driving, Two Important Papers," *Ophthalmic Optician,* Vol. 7, No. 2, Jan. 1967, 73–79.

DAVID, J. H., and LARRY LETT. "Study of the Effect of Using Colored Guide Posts in

Interstate Highways to Reduce Accidental Damage," Alabama State Highway Department (Montgomery, Ala. 36104), HPR Report No. 33, Aug. 1968, 22 pp.

DAVIS, ADELLE. *Let's Get Well*, Harcourt, Brace, & World, New York, 1965.

DAWSON. Report of Department of Transportation Act: H.R. 1701, Washington, D. C., House of Representatives of Eighty-ninth Congress, Second Session, 1966.

DAWSON, NOEL K. "Too Dangerous to Drive," *Popular Mechanics*, Vol. 127, No. 1, Jan. 1967, 99–101, 212.

DEMOTT, D. W., and R. M BOYNTON. "Retinal Distribution of Entoptic Stray Light," *Journal of the Optical Society of America*, Vol. 48, 1958, 13.

Department of Scientific and Industrial Research. *Research on Road Safety*, Her Majesty's Stationery Office, London, 1963.

———. *Dipped Headlights Campaigns in 1963–64*, Road Research Technical Paper No. 73, Her Majesty's Stationery Office, London, 1964.

———. *Use of Headlamps*, Working Party on the Lighting of Motor Vehicles, Report to the Minister of Transport, Her Majesty's Stationery Office, London, 1967.

"Designing the 100 MPH Expressway," *Highway Research News*, No. 34, Winter 1969, 48–52.

"Doctors 'Prescribe' for Highway Safety," *Traffic Safety*, Vol. 65, No. 11, Nov. 1965, 16.

DOMEY, RICHARD G. "Flicker Fusion, Dark Adaptation and Age as Predictors of Night Vision," *Highway Research Board Bulletin* 336, Jan. 1962, 22–25.

———. "Predictors of Night Vision," *Proceedings, Symposium on Visibility in the Driving Task*, sponsored by Highway Research Board, Illuminating Engineering Research Institute, and Texas A & M University, May 13–15, 1968, 69–74.

———, and ROSS A. MCFARLAND. "Dark Adaptation as a Function of Age: Individual Prediction," *American Journal of Ophthalmology*, Vol. 51, No. 6, 1961, 1262–1268.

———, and ———. "Operator and Vehicle Design," *Human Factors in Technology*, E. M. Bennett, J. Degan, and J. Spiegel, eds., McGraw-Hill, New York, 1963.

———, ———, and ERNEST CHADWICK. "Threshold and Rate of Dark Adaptation as Functions of Age and Time," *Human Factors*, Vol. 2, No. 3, 1960, 109–119.

———, ———, and ———. "Dark Adaptation as a Function of Age, II," *Journal of Gerontology*, Vol. 15, No. 3, July 1960, 267–279.

"Drinking Drivers at Fault in One Half of Auto Deaths," *Highway Research Abstracts*, Vol. 36, No. 11, Nov. 1966, 14.

"Driver Behavior," *Proceedings of the Second Annual Traffic Safety Research Symposium of the Automobile Insurance Industry*, Insurance Institute for Highway Safety (Suite 711, Watergate Office Bldg., 2600 Virginia Ave. NW, Washington, D.C., 20037).

"Drivers' Medical Screening Urged," *AMA News*, March 21, 1966, 1.

"Drivers' Vision and Car Design," *Optician*, May 3, 1963, 445.

DUREMAN, INGMAR, et al. "A Dose Response Study of Diazepam (Valium) and 4306 CB (Tranxilen) During Prolonged Simulated Car Driving," Department of Psychology, University of Uppsala, Sweden, Report 54, Sept. 1968.

EASTMAN, A. A., S. K. GUTH, and G. A. BRECHER. "Instrument with Variable Beam Splitter for Measuring Contrast Sensitivity," *Investigative Ophthalmology*, Vol. 2, Feb. 1963, 37–46.

"Effect of Glare on Drivers' Vision," *Ophthalmic Optician*, April 2, 1966, 363.

ELLIOTT, F. R., and C. M. LOUTTIT. "Auto Braking Reaction Time to Visual vs. Auditory Warning Signals," *Proceedings of the Indiana Academy of Sciences*, Vol. 47, 1937, 220–225.

ELSTAD, J. O., J. T. FITZPATRICK, and H. L. WOLTMAN. "Requisite Luminance Characteristics for Reflective Signs," *Highway Research Board Bulletin 336*, Jan. 1962, 51–60.

ENGELKING, E. "Die Tritanomalie, ein bisher unbekannter Typus Anomaler Trichromasie," *Albrecht von Graefe's Archiv für Ophthalmologie*, Vol. 116, 1925, 196.

"Environment: Visual Effects of the Atmosphere," *Visual Factors in Automobile Driving*, Stanley S. Ballard, and Henry A. Knoll, eds., Highway Research Board of the National Academy of Sciences-National Academy of Engineering, Washington, D.C., 1958, 6.

ERCOLES, A. M. "On the Recovery of Sensitivity Subsequent to Either White or Yellow Glare," *Atti Fond Ronchi*, Vol. 15, 1960, 164–271.

EVANS, J. N., and Ross A. McFARLAND. "Effects of Oxygen Deprivation on the Central Visual Field," *American Journal of Ophthalmology*, Vol. 21, no. 9, 1938, 968–980.

Factors Influencing Safety at Highway-Rail Grade Crossings, National Cooperative Highway Research Program Report 50, National Research Council, National Academy of Sciences-National Academy of Engineering, Alan M. Voorhees & Associates, McLean, Va., 1968.

FAULKNER, C. R., and S. J. OLDER. "Effects of Different Systems of Vehicle Lighting on a Driver's Ability to See Dark Objects in Well-lit Streets," *Road Research Laboratory, Ministry of Transport* Report LR113, Crowthorne, 1967.

Federal Government of Canada, Brief on Traffic Accident Deaths and Injuries in Canada, Ottawa, 1965.

"Federal Specifications and Standards: Standard Safety Devices for Automotive Vehicles," *Federal Register*, Vol. 30, No. 125, June 1965, 8319.

FELDHAUS, J. L., JR. "Dynamic Visual Acuity—Effect on Night Driving and Highway Accidents," *Highway Research Board Bulletin 298*, Washington, D.C., 1961.

FERGUSON, H. H. "Road Accidents: Pedestrians' Beliefs Regarding Visibility at Night," *Journal of Applied Psychology*, Vol. 28, 1944, 109–116.

————, and W. R. GEDDES. "A Dangerous Pedestrian Belief," *Road Accidents*, Psychological Laboratory, University of Otago, New Zealand (the experiment described was carried out in July 1939), 199–205.

FILDERMAN, IRVING P. "Clinical Procedure for Adapting the Telecon Lens," *Journal of the American Optometric Association*, Vol. 30, No. 8, March 1959, 561–562.

FINCH, D. M., "Factors Influencing Night Visibility of Roadway Obstacles," *Illuminating Engineering*, Vol. 51, 1956.

————. "Roadway Delineation with Curb Marker Lights," *Highway Research Board Bulletin 336*, 1962, 105–109.

FINE, JEROME L., "Development of a Criterion for Driver Behavior," *Highway Research Abstracts*, Vol. 36, No. 6, June 1966, 4.

FISHER, A. J. "Photometric Specification for Vehicular Traffic Signal Lanterns, Part I," Institute of Highway and Traffic Research, University of New South Wales, Kensington, Australia, Feb, 1969.

————, and CHRISTIE, A. W. "Note on Disability Glare," *Vision Research*, Vol. 5, 1965, 565–571.

————, and A. B. CROUCH. "Measurement of Coloured Lights of High Luminance Using a Spectra Pritchard Photometer," *Australian Road Research*, Vol. 3, No. 7, 1968, 21–24.

FISHER, R. L., "Accident and Operating Experience at Interchanges," *Highway Research Bulletin 291*, 126.

"Fitness to Drive Motor Vehicles," *Optician*, Vol. 136, 1960, 666–668.

FITZPATRICK, J. T. "Uniform Reflective Sign, Pavement and Delineation Treatments for Night Traffic Guidance," *Highway Research Board Bulletin 255*, 1960, 138–145.

FLOM, MERTON C. "Prognosis in Strabismus," *American Journal of Optometry and Archives of the American Academy of Optometry*, Vol. 35, No. 10, 1958, 509–514.

"Fog Surrounding the Fog Problem Being Swept Away by N.J.'s Unique Nylon Broom," *Highway Research News*, 5.

FOLDVARY, L. A. "Effect of Compulsory Safety Helmets on Motorcycle Accident Fatalities," *Australian Road Research*, Vol. 2, Sept. 1964, 9.

————. "Analysis of Age and Experience of Responsible and Non-Responsible Drivers Involved in Motorcycle vs. Other Motor Vehicle Collisions in Victoria, 1961 and 1962," *Australian Road Research*, Vol. 2, No. 3, March 1965, 48.

FORBES, T. W. "Psychological Applications to the New Field of Traffic Engineering," *Journal of Applied Psychology*, Vol. 25, No. 1, Feb. 1941, 52–58.

————. "Driver Characteristics and Highway Operation," *Traffic Engineering*, Nov. 1953.

————. "Some Factors Affecting Driver Efficiency at Night," *Highway Research Board Bulletin 255*, 1960, 66.

————. "Driver Behavior Requirements and Discovering Deficiencies," *Optometric Weekly*, Vol. 51, 1960, 2556–2558.

————. "Human Factors in Highway Design, Operation and Safety Problems," *Human Factors*, Vol. 2, Feb., 1960, 1–3.

————. "Study of Accident Hazard in Relation to Fenders and Mudguards for Motor Vehicles," *Traffic Safety Research Review*, Vol. 6, No. 1, 1962, 16–19.

————. "Predicting Attention-Gaining Characteris ics of Highway Traffic Signs: Measurement Technique," *Human Factors*, Aug. 1964, 371–374.

————. "Traffic Engineers and Driver Behavior," *Traffic Safety Research Review*, Vol. 9, No. 3, Sept. 1965, 87–89.

————, K. MOSCOWITZ, and G. MORGAN. "A Comparison of Lower Case and Capital Letters for Highway Signs," *Proceedings of the Thirteenth Annual Meeting of the Highway Research Board*, 1950, 355–377.

————, and M. S. KATZ. "Summary of Human Engineering Research Data and Principles Related to Highway Design and Traffic Engineering Problems," American Institute for Research, Pittsburgh, April 1957.

————, et al. "Measurement of Driver Reactions to Tunnel Condition," *Highway Research Board Proceedings*, Vol. 37, 1958, 345–357.

————, E. GERVAIS, and T. ALLEN. "Effectiveness of Symbols for Lane Control Signals," Michigan State University, Highway Traffic Safety Center and Michigan State Highway Department, East Lansing, Dec. 1958.

————, T. E. SNYDER, and R. F. PAIN. *A Study of Traffic Sign Requirements: An Annotated Bibliography*, East Lansing, Mich., 1964.

————, ————, and ————. "Traffic Sign Requirements," *Highway Research Board Bulletin 70*, 1963 and 1964, ten reports.

————, et al. "Low Contrast and Standard Visual Acuity under Mesopic and Photopic Illumination," Highway Traffic Safety Center and Department of Psychology, Michigan State University (East Lansing), Dec. 1967.

————, et al. "Letter and Sign Contrast, Brightness, and Size Effects on Visibility," *Highway Research Board Bulletin 216*, 1968, 48–54.

————, et al. "Color and Brightness Factors in Simulated and Full-Scale Traffic Sign Visibility," *Highway Research Board Bulletin 216*, 1968, 55–65.

FORD, RICHARD, and ALFRED L. MOSELEY. "Motor Vehicle Suicides," Highway Research Abstracts, Vol. 33, No. 6, June 1963, 14.

FORD, HENRY, II. "Henry Ford II Talks About Car Safety," *Popular Science*, Vol. 187, No. 6, Dec. 1965, 62–65.

FORNEY, ROBERT B. "Combined Effect of Ethanol and Other Drugs," *Prevention of Highway Injury*, Selzer, Gikas, and Huelke, eds., Highway Safety Research Institute, University of Michigan (Ann Arbor), 1967, 70.

FORTUIN, G. J. *Visual Power and Visibility* (Rijks-Universteit of Groningen, The Netherlands), Doctoral Dissertation, 1951.

FOSBERRY, R. A. C., and R. L. MOORE. "Vision From the Driver's Seat," reprint of paper to JIDITVA Conference on Technical Inspection of Motor Vehicles, Brussels, by Motor Industry Research Association, England, 1963.

FOX, PHYLLIS, and FREDERICK LEHMAN. *Computer Simulation of Single Lane Automobile Traffic*, Newark, 1965.

FRY, GLENN A. "Re-evaluation of the Scattering Theory of Glare," *Illuminating Engineering*, Vol. 49, 1954, 98.

————. "Relation of the Configuration of a Brightness Contrast Border to Its Visibility," *Journal of the Optical Society of America*, Vol. 37, 1947, 166.

————. "Assessment of Visual Performances," *Illuminating Engineering*, Vol. 57, No. 6, 1962.

————. "Transient Adaptation of the Eyes of a Motorist," *Highway Research Board Bulletin 366*, 1962, 110.

————. "Visual Performance Under Varying States of Adaptation," *Proceedings, Symposium on Visibility in the Driving Task*, sponsored by Highway Research Board, Illuminating Engineering Research Institute, and Texas A & M University, May 13–15, 1968, 96–105.

———, and P. W. COBB. "Visual Discrimination of Two Parallel Bright Bars in a Dark Field," *American Journal of Psychology*, Vol. 49, 1937, 265.

———, B. S. PRITCHARD, and H. R. BLACKWELL. "Design and Calibration of a Disability Glare Lens," *Illuminating Engineering*, Vol. 58, 120–123, 1963.

GALLAWAY, BOB M. "Skid Resistance and Polishing Type Aggregates," *Texas Transportation Researcher*, Vol. 5, No. 1, Jan. 1969, 3–7.

GARRETT, JOHN W. *Ocular Orbital Injuries in Automobile Crashes*, Bulletin No. 4, Automobile Crash Injury Research, Cornell Aeronautical Laboratory, March 1963.

GASSON, A. P., and G. S. PETERS. "Effect of Concentration Upon the Apparent Size of the Visual Field in Binocular Vision" (student research project under direction of Prof. J. B. DAVEY, London), *Optician*, Jan. 1, and 8, 1965.

GERATHEWOHL, S. J. "Conspicuity of Steady and Flashing Light Signals: Variation of Contrast," *Journal of the Optical Society of America*, Vol. 43, No. 7, July 1953, 567–571.

GIBSON, J. J. "Motion Picture Testing and Research," U.S. Army Air Force Aviation Psychology Program, Research Report No. 7, 1946, 62.

GIBSON, JACK R. "Visibility: A Bibliography" (2,100 references), Library of Congress Technical Information Division, Washington, D.C., 1952.

GIOIA, ANTHONY J., and CLARENCE MORPHEW. "Evaluation of Driver Vision," Proceedings of General Motors Corp. Automotive Safety Seminar, July 11–12, 1968, Paper No. 10. General Motors Proving Ground (Milford, Mich. 48042), 14 pp.

"Glass in New Car Reacts to Light," *New York Times*, Nov. 28, 1965.

"GM Experiments with New Road-Vehicle Communications System Dubbed 'Dair,'" *Highway Research News*, No. 24, Summer 1966, 33–35.

GOLDBERG, L. "Quantitative Studies on Alcohol Tolerance in Man," *Acta Physiologica Scandinavica*, Vol. 5, 1943.

———. "Alcohol Induced Nystagmus," *Alcohol and Road Traffic*, Proceedings of 3rd International Conference, B.M.A. House, London, 1963.

GOLDSMITH, JOHN R., and STEPHEN A. LANDAW. "Carbon Monoxide and Human Health," *Science*, Vol. 162, No. 3860, Dec. 20, 1968, 1352–1359.

GOLDSTEIN, A. G. "Linear Acceleration and Apparent Distance," *Perceptual and Motor Skills*, Vol. 9, 1959, 267–269.

GOLDSTEIN, LEON G. *Research on Human Variables in Safe Motor Vehicle Operation: A Correlational Summary of Predictor Variables and Criterion Measures*, George Washington University, Washington, D.C., 1961.

———. *Human Variables in Traffic Accidents*, National Academy of Sciences–National Research Council, Washington, D.C., 1962.

GONSETH, A. T. "Effectiveness of Holland Tunnel Transitional Lighting During the Winter Months," *Highway Research Board Bulletin 255*, 1960, 79–91.

GOODWIN, H., et al. "Investigation of the Effects of Ethyl Alcohol on Visual Functions," paper presented before the American Academy of Optometry, Denver, Dec. 1966.

GORDON, DONALD A. *Experimental Isolation of the Driver's Visual Input*, U. S. Department of Commerce, Bureau of Public Roads, Washington, D.C.

———. "Static and Dynamic Visual Fields in Human Space Perception," *Journal of the Optical Society of America*, Vol. 55, No. 10, Oct. 1965.

GRAMBERG-DANIELSON, B. "Ursachen des Pulfrich Phenomens und seine Bedeutung im Strassenverkehr," *Klinische Monatsblätter für Augenheilkunde*, Vol. 142, 1963, 738.

———. "Das Sehen im Strassenverkehr," *Klinisch Monatsblätter für Augenheilkunde*, Vol. 143, 1964.

GREENSHIELDS, B. D. and F. N. PLATT. "Driver Behavior Study," Aug. 1961, quoting *Traffic Engineering* by Matson, Smith, and Hurd, McGraw-Hill, 1955.

———, and ———. "Driver Behavior Study," University of Michigan Transportation Institute, Aug. 1961.

———, and ———. "Objective Measurements of Driver Behavior," Paper 809A presented at SAE Automotive Engineering Congress, Detroit, Jan. 1964.

GREY, MICHEL. "Road User and the Improvement of Vehicle Registration Plates," *In-*

ternational Police Chronicle, No. 70, Jan.-Feb. 1965, 8–20.

GRIME, G. *Crompton-Lanchester Lecture: Automobile Lighting and Visibility*, Institution of Mechanical Engineers, England, 1960.

———. "Car Design and Operation in Relation to Road Safety," *Practioner*, Vol. 188, April 1962, 447–456.

———, and R. D. LISTER. *Inspection of Vehicles for Road Worthiness with Special Reference to Methods and Equipment*, Road Research Laboratory, Harmondsworth, Middlesex, Eng., 1957.

GRINDLEY, G. C. "Notes on the Perception of Movement in Relation to the Problem of Landing an Aeroplane," WAM-100-15, FPRC 426, March 1942.

GUERRY, DU PONT. "Ophthalmological Aspects of Driver Licensing and Repeat Offenses," *Journal of the American Medical Association*, Jan. 26, 1957, 227–228.

GUTH, SHERMAN L. "The Effect of Wavelength on Visual Perception Latency," *Vision Research*, Vol. 4, Dec. 1964, 567–578.

GUTH, SYLVESTER K. "Effects of Age on Visibility," *American Journal of Optometry and Archives of American Academy of Optometry*, Vol. 34, No. 9, 1957, 463–477.

———. "Method for the Evaluation of Discomfort Glare," *Illumination Engineering*, Vol. 58, No. 5, May 1963, 351–364.

———, and ARTHUR A. EASTMAN. "Brightness Difference in Seeing," *American Journal of Optometry and Archives of American Academy of Optometry*, Monograph No. 169, Nov. 1954.

HABER, HEINZ. "Safety Hazard of Tinted Automobile Windshields at Night," *Journal of the Optical Society of America*, Vol. 45, No. 6, June 1955, 413–419.

HADDON, WILLIAM, JR. "Changing Approach to the Epidemiology, Prevention, and Amelioration of Trauma: The Transition to Approaches Etiologically Rather Than Descriptively Based," Presented at the 95th Annual Meeting of the American Public Health Association, program on Epidemiology of Traffic Accidents, Miami Beach, Fla., Oct. 26, 1967.

———, EDWARD A. SUCHMAN, and DAVID KLEIN. *Accident Research*, Harper and Row, New York, 1964.

———, *et al.* "Controlled Investigation of the Characteristics of Adult Pedestrians Fatally Injured by Motor Vehicles in Manhattan," *Journal of Chronic Diseases*, Vol. 14, 1961, 655–678.

HAIGHT, FRANK A. "Traffic Death and Suicide: A Statistical Study," Institute of Transportation and Traffic Engineering, University of California (Berkeley), Special Report, 1965, 38 pp.

HALPERIN, MEYER H., *et al.* "Time Course of the Effects of Carbon Monoxide on Visual Thresholds," *Journal of Physiology*, Vol. 146, No. 3, 1959, 583–593.

HARE, CHARLES T., and ROBERT H. HEMION. *Headlight Beam Usage on U.S. Highways*, Project No. 11-1908, Final Report on Phase III of a Study for the Bureau of Public Roads, Federal Highway Administration, U.S. Department of Transportation under U.S. Contract No. 11-4126, Southwest Research Institute, San Antonio, Tex., Dec. 2, 1968.

HARRINGTON, T. L., and McRAE K. JOHNSON. "Improved Instrument for Measurement of Pavement Marking Reflective Performance," *Highway Research Board Bulletin 336*, 1962, 111–113.

HARRIS, A. J. *Vehicle Headlighting: Visibility and Glare*, Department of Scientific and Industrial Research, London, 1954.

HARTMANN, E. "Disability Glare and Discomfort Glare," in Eric Ingelstam, ed., *Lighting Problems in Highway Traffic*, Macmillan Co., New York, 1963, 95–109.

———. "Die Blendung aus der Sicht des Physikers," *Berichte der Deutschen Ophthalmologischen Gesellschaft in Heidelberg*, Vol. 65, 1963, 446.

———. "Threshold of Disability Glare," *Highway Research Abstracts*, Vol. 34, No. 7, July 1964, 12.

Harvard School of Public Health. "Human Factors in Highway Transport Safety" (description of research reports), 1955 (4).

HAVENS, JAMES H. and ALLIE C. PEED, JR. "Spherical Lens Optics Applied to Retrodirective Reflection," *Highway Research Board Bulletin 56*, 1952, 66–77.

HEAD, J., *et al. Pedestrian Traffic Accidents Involving Children in the City of Vancouver, Canada,* University of British Columbia, Vancouver, 1963.

HEATH, GORDON G. "Luminosity Curves of Normal and Dichromatic Observers," *Science,* Vol. 128, 1958, 775.

————, and INGEBORG SCHMIDT. "Signal Color Recognition by Color Defective Observers," *American Journal of Optometry and Archives of American Academy of Optometry,* Vol. 36, No. 8, Aug. 1959, 421–437.

HEATH, WARREN M., and DAN M. FITCH. "Determination of Windshield Levels Requisite for Driving Visibility," *Highway Research Board Bulletin 56,* 1952, 1–16.

HECHT, S., and C. G. MULLER. "Visibility of Lines and Squares at High Brightness," *Journal of the Optical Society of America,* Vol. 37, 1947, 500.

HECHT, S., and E. U. MINTZ. "Visibility of Single Lines at Various Illuminations and the Retinal Basis of Visual Resolution," *Journal of General Physiology,* Vol. 22, 1939, 593.

HEINSEN, ARTHUR C., JR. *Reflectorized License Plates: Their Advantages,* San Jose, Calif., 1965.

HEMION, ROGER H. "Glare Factor on Two-Lane Highways," *Proceedings, Symposium on Visibility in the Driving Task,* sponsored by Highway Research Board, Illuminating Engineering Research Institute, and Texas A & M University, May 13–15, 1968, 145–146.

————. "Effect of Headlight Glare on Vehicle Control and Detection of Highway Vision Targets," Project No. 11-1908, Southwest Research Institute, San Antonio, Tex.

HENDERSON, HAROLD L., and ANGELO DISPENZIERI. *Automobility: Adding a New Dimension to Total Physical Rehabilitation,* Drivers Safety Service, New York, N.Y., 1964.

HERBERT, EVAN. "Traffic Safety," *International Science and Technology* (205 E. 42nd St., New York, N.Y.), Sept. 1966.

HERMAN, R., *et al.* "Traffic Dynamics: Analysis of Stability in Car Following," *Operations Research,* Vol. 6, No. 2, March-April 1958; Vol. 7, No. 1, Jan.-Feb. 1959.

————, and K. GARDELS. "Vehicular Traffic Flow," *Scientific American,* Vol. 209, No. 6, Dec. 1963.

HERRINGTON, C. G. "Design of Reflectorized Motor Vehicle License Plates," *Highway Research Board Proceedings,* Vol. 39, 1960, 441–466.

HESS, E. H., and J. M. POLT. "Pupil Size as Related to Interest Value of Visual Stimuli," *Science,* Vol. 132, 1960, 349–350.

HICKS, CLIFFORD B., and MERRILL J. ALLEN. "Are You an Invisible Driver?" *Popular Mechanics,* Vol. 122, No. 5, Nov. 1964, 114–117.

Highway Research Board. *Bibliography—Night Visibility, Selected References,* National Academy of Sciences–National Academy of Engineering, No. 45, 1967.

————. *Proceedings, Symposium on Visibility in the Driving Task,* sponsored by Highway Research Board, Illuminating Engineering Research Institute, and Texas A and M University, May 13–15, 1968.

————. *Highway Research Record No. 216, Lighting, Visibility, and Driving, 6 Reports,* National Academy of Sciences–National Academy of Engineering, 1968.

Highway Safety, Design and Operations: Roadside Hazards, Hearings before the Special Subcommittee on the Federal-Aid Highway Program of the Committee on Public Works, House of Representatives, Ninetieth Congress, U.S. Government Printing Office, Washington, 1968.

HILDEBRAND, G., and H. WAKELAND. *Feasibility Study, New York State Safety Car Program, Final Report,* Fairchild Hiller, Republic Aviation Division, Farmingdale, L.I., N.Y., 1966.

HILL, N. E. G. "Recognition of Colored Light Signals Which Are Near the Limit of Visibility," *Proceedings, Physical Society* (London), Vol. 59, 1947, 560–574.

HIRSCH, MONROE, and RALPH E. WICK. *Vision of the Aging Patient,* Chilton Co., Philadelphia, 1960, xviii and 328.

HOCKENBEAMER, E. F. "Side Vision Versus Speed," Claims and Safety Department, Pacific Gas and Electric Co., San Francisco, Calif., 1952.

HOFER, RUDOLPH, JR. "Glare Screen for Divided Highways," *Highway Research Board Bulletin 336,* Jan. 1962, 95–101.

HOFFMAN, ERROL R., and PETER N. JOUBERT. "Effect of Changes in Some Vehicle Handling Variables on Driver Steering Performance," *Human Factors,* Vol. 8, No. 3, June 1966, 245–263.

HOFSTETTER, HENRY W. "Illumination for Sight Testing," *Illuminating Engineering,* Vol. 46, No. 3, March 1951, 116–118.

————. *Industrial Vision,* Chilton Co., Philadelphia, 1956.

————. "Visual Performance Following Optometric Correction," *Optica International,* Vol. 3, No. 2, June 1966, 46–51.

————. "Computed Distances of Legibility of Standard Traffic Control Signs," *Journal of the American Optometric Association,* Vol. 38, No. 5, May 1967, 381–385.

————. "Alpascope, An Instrument Review," *Journal of the American Optometric Association,* Vol. 39, No. 1, Jan. 1968.

————, and LOWELL B. ZERBE. "Prevalence of 20/20 with Best, Previous, and No Lens Correction," *Journal of the American Optometric Association,* Vol. 29, No. 12, July 1958, 772-774.

————, and W. M. LYLE. "Modification of the Bio-Photometer for Alterocular Fixation Control," *Highway Research Board Bulletin 336, Night Visibility,* 1962, National Academy of Sciences–National Research Council publication 1018; also in *American Journal of Optometry and Archives of American Academy of Optometry,* Vol. 40, No. 1, Jan. 1963, 35–40.

————, and R. READING. "Extra Horopteral Stereopsis in Vehicle Operator Orientation," *Highway Research News,* No. 17, Feb. 1965, 84–90.

HOLLADAY, L. L. "Fundamentals of Glare and Visibility," *Journal of the Optical Society of America,* Vol. 12, 1926, 271.

HON, CONRAD C., JR. "Headlight Glare Solved by Rearward Directed Fender Mounted Side Light," personal correspondence to Senator Abraham A. Ribicoff from 521 Old Bridge Road, Northport, L.I., N.Y., Nov. 1955.

HONEGGER, VON H., and W. D. SCHAFER. "Sehscharfe für bewegte Objekte Einige Gesichtspunkte für die Verkehrmedizin," *Zentralblatt für Verkehrs-Medizin, Verkehrs-Psychologie, Luft-und Raumfahrt-Medizin,* Vol. 14, No. 1968, 160–167.

HOPKIN, V. D. "A Selective Review of Peripheral Vision," *Great Britain Flying Personnel Research Commission,* Vol. 1128, 1959.

HOPKINSON, R. G., and R. C. BRADLEY. "Study of Glare from Very Large Sources," *Illuminating Engineering,* Vol. 55, 1960, 288–294.

HOPPE, DONALD A., and A. R. LAUER. "Factors Affecting the Perception of Relative Motion and Distance Between Vehicles at Night," *Studies in Night Visibility,* Highway Research Board, Washington, D.C., 1951, 11–16.

HOUGHTON, H. G. "On the Relation Between Visibility and the Constitution of Clouds and Fog," *Journal of Aeronautical Sciences,* Vol. 6, 1939, 408–411.

————, and W. H. RADFORD. "On the Measurement of Drop-size and Liquid Water Content in Fogs and Clouds," *Papers in Physiological Oceanography and Meteorology* (Cambridge, Mass.), Vol. 6, No. 4, 1938.

————, and W. R. CHALKER. "Scattering Cross Section of Water Drops in Air for Visible Light," *Journal of the Optical Society of America,* Vol. 39, No. 11, Nov. 1949, 955–957.

HOWARD, J., and D. M. FINCH. "Visual Characteristics of Flashing Roadway Hazard Warning Devices," *Highway Research Board Bulletin 255,* 1960, 146–157.

HOWELL, W. C., and G. E. BRIGGS. "Effects of Visual Noise and Locus of Perturbation on Tracking Performance," *Journal of Experimental Psychology,* Vol. 58, 1959, 166–173, from *Aerospace Medicine,* Vol. 331, 1960, A8.

HUBER, MATTEW J. "Traffic Operations and Driver Performance as Related to Various Conditions of Nighttime Visibility," *Highway Research Board Bulletin 336,* 1962, 37–50.

HULBERT, SLADE F. "Signing a Freeway to Freeway Interchange (Guide Signs)," Institute of Transportation and Traffic Engineering, University of California (Los Angeles), Sept. 1965, 1–19.

————, *et al.* "Preliminary Study of Dynamic Visual Acuity and its Effect in Motorists' Vision," *Journal of the American Optometric Association,* Vol. 29, 1958, 359–364.

————, and ALBERT BURG. "Effects of Underlining on the Readability of Highway Destination Signs," *Highway Research Board Proceedings,* Vol. 36, 1957, 561–574.

————, and JINX BEERS. "Wrong Way Driving Off-Ramp Studies," Institute of Transportation and Traffic Engineering, University of California (Los Angeles), Dec. 1966, 1–16.

HUTCHINSON, JOHN. "Planning for Highway Safety," *Research Review,* Vol. 9, No. 3, Sept. 1965, 83–86.

HYDE, W. LEWIS. "Periscopes for Rear Vision," Paper No. 680403, Society of Automotive Engineers Mid-Year Meeting, Detroit, May 20–24, 1968.

"Illumination," *Traffic Control and Roadway Elements* (Report of the Automotive Safety Foundation and the U.S. Bureau of Public Roads), 1963, 77–79.

Indiana State Police. *Indiana State Police Auto Crash Injury Research,* 3d ed., Indianapolis, Ind., 1957.

Indiana University. *Role of the Drinking Driver in Traffic Accidents* (Grand Rapids study), Department of Police Administration, Bloomington, Ind., 1964.

Industrial Medical Association. *Medical Aspects of Driver Licensing,* 1964.

INGELSTAM, ERIK, ed., *Lighting Problems in Highway Traffic,* Pergamon Press, London, 1963.

Institute for Perception. *Studies in Perception,* dedicated to M. A. Bouman, RVO-TNO, National Defense Research Organization, TNO, Soesterberg, The Netherlands, 1966.

Institute of Traffic Engineers. "Freeway Operations," report of Freeway Operations Seminars.

Insurance Institute for Highway Safety. "Driver Behavior," Proceedings Second Annual Traffic Safety Research Symposium of the Automobile Insurance Industry (Suite 711, Watergate Office Bldg., 2600 Virginia Ave. NW, Washington, D.C. 20037), March 1968.

International Federation of Pedestrians. *Voice of the Pedestrian,* April 1968.

International Organization for Standardization. "Driver's Daylight Goggles, Draft Proposal," Institute Für Medizin Optik, Universitat München (Barbara Strasse, 16).

IRLAND, M. J., and V. L. LINDBERG. "Control of Double Images in Automobile Glass," Paper No. 650536, Society of Automotive Engineers Mid-Year Meeting, Chicago, May 1965.

IRVIN, ROBERT. "Will Cars Ever Be Safer?" *Louisville Courier-Journal Supplement,* March 6, 1966.

JAYLE, GAËTAN E., et al. *Night Vision,* Charles C. Thomas, Springfield, Ill., Vol. 14, 1959.

JELLINEK, E. M., and ROSS A. McFARLAND. "Analysis of Psychological Experiments on the Effects of Alcohol," *Quarterly Journal of Studies on Alcohol,* Vol. 1, No. 2, 1940, 272–371.

JOHANSSON, GUNNAR, F. BACKLUND, and S. S. BERGSTROM. *Studies in Motion Thresholds,* Psychological Laboratory, University of Uppsala, Sweden, Reports 1 and 2, Nov. 1957.

————, and F. BACKLUND. *An Eye Movement Recorder,* Psychological Laboratory, University of Uppsala, Sweden, Report 8, 1960.

————, et al. *Visible Distances During Night Driving,* Psychological Laboratory, University of Uppsala, Sweden, Report 9, Aug. 1961.

————. *Perception of Motion and Changing Form,* Psychological Laboratory, University of Uppsala, Sweden, Report 10, Oct. 1963.

————, et al. *Drivers and Road Signs I,* Psychological Laboratory, University of Uppsala, Sweden, Report 11, Nov. 1963.

————, and CHRIS OTTANDER. *Light Adaptation and Glare,* Psychological Laboratory, University of Uppsala, Sweden, Report 12, Nov. 1963.

————, and KARE RUMAR. *Available Braking Distances in Night Driving,* Psychological Laboratory, University of Uppsala, Sweden, Report 13, Nov. 1963.

————, and ————. *Silhouette Effects in Night Driving,* Psychological Laboratory, University of Uppsala, Sweden, Report 19, Nov. 1964.

————, and ————. *Drivers' Brake-Reaction Times,* Psychological Laboratory, University of Uppsala, Sweden, Report 26, March 1965.

————, and ————. "Drivers and Road Signs: A Preliminary Investigation of the Capacity of Car Drivers to Get Information from Road Signs," *Ergonomics,* Vol. 9, No. 1, 1966, 57.

———, and ———. "Visible Distances and Safe Approach Speeds for Night Driving," *Ergonomics,* Vol. 11, No. 3, 1968, 275–282.

———, and FREDERIK BACKLUND. *Drivers and Road Signs II,* Psychological Laboratory, University of Uppsala, Sweden, Report 50, April 1968.

JOST, F. "Tabakrauchen und Strassenverkehr" (Tobacco Smoking and Street Traffic), *Medizinische Welt,* No. 1, Jan. 1965, 30–35.

JUDD, DEANE B. "Facts of Color-Blindness," *J.O.S.A.,* Vol. 33, No. 6, June 1943, 294–307.

KARMEIER, D. F., C. G. HERRINGTON, and J. E. BAERWALD. "Comprehensive Analysis of Motor Vehicle License Plates," *Highway Research Board Proceedings,* Vol. 39, 1960, 416–440.

KEARNEY, PAUL W. *Drivers' Eye Tests: A Nation-Wide Farce,* American Optometric Association, St. Louis, Mo., 1959.

———. *Highway Homicide,* Thomas Y. Crowell Co., New York, 1966.

KERRICK, J. C. "A Discussion of Current Driver Licensing Practices," *Journal of the American Optometric Association,* Vol. 32, 1960, 224–236.

KING, J. N. "Measurement of Driver Visibility," *Optician,* Vol. 139, 1960, 110–112.

KING, LEE ELLIS, and ERNEST C. CURWEN. *Visibility of Colored Lights in Dense Fog,* delivered before 45th Annual Meeting, Highway Research Board, Washington, D.C., Jan. 1966.

———, and D. M. FINCH. "Daytime Running Lights," *Highway Research Record 275,* 1969.

KINNEY, J. A. S., E. J. SWEENY, and A. P. RYAN. "A New Night Vision Sensitivity Test," *A.F. Medical Journal,* Vol. 11, 1960, 1020–1029.

———, and M. M. CONNORS. "Recovery of Foveal Dark Adaptation," *Highway Research Record 70,* 1965, 35.

KITE, C. R., and J. N. KING. "Survey of the Factors Limiting the Visual Fields of Motor Vehicle Drivers in Relation to Minimum Visual Field and Visibility Standards," *British Journal of Physiological Optics,* Vol. 18, April 1961, 85–107.

KNOLL, H. A. "A Brief History of 'Nocturnal Myopia' and Related Phenomena," *American Journal of Optometry and Archives of American Academy of Optometry,* Vol. 29, No. 2, 1952, 69–81.

———. "Effect of Low Levels of Luminance and Freedom from Optical Stimulation of Accommodation Upon the Refractive State of the Eye," Armed Forces NRC Vision Committee, Minutes of 31st Meeting, Nov. 20–22, 1952.

KONIG, A., and C. DIETERICI. "Die Grundempfindungen in Normalen und Anomalen Farbensystemen und Ihre Intensitatsverteilung im Spektrum," *Zeitschrift für Psychologie,* Vol. 4, 1893, 241.

KRIES, J. V. "Ueber Farbensysteme," *Zeitschrift für Psychologie,* Vol. 13, 1897, 239, 268, 315.

KUZIOMKO, LOUISE M., and BASIL Y. SCOTT. "Upgrading Driver Licensing Vision Re-Examination," *Traffic Digest and Review* (1804 Hinman Ave., Evanston, Ill., 60204), Vol. 16, No. 8, Aug. 1968, 14–19.

LAUER, A. R. "History and Development of the Driving Research Laboratory," *Optometric Weekly,* March 20, 1947.

———. "What Visual Acuity Is Needed for Night Driving?" *Optometric Weekly,* Vol. 41, 1950, 485–488.

———. "Certain Factors Influencing the Tolerance of Light and Visual Acuity," study carried out in the Engineering Experiment Station at Iowa State College, project of Committee on Motorists' Vision of the American Optometric Association.

———. *Psychology of Driving, Factors of Traffic Enforcement,* Charles C Thomas, Springfield, Ill., 1960, xxvii and 324.

———, and H. KOTVIS. "Automotive Manipulation in Relation to Vision," *Journal of Applied Psychology,* Vol. 18, 1934, 422–431.

———, and EDWIN H. SILVER. "Survey of Research on Night Driving in Relation to Vision," a study made by the Engineering Experiment Station at Iowa State College in cooperation with the American Optometric Association.

LAVENDER, H. JERRY, JR., and RAYMOND M. EKSTROM. "Red-Green Paradox," *Human Factors,* Vol. 10, No. 1, 1968, 63–66.

LEBENSOHN, JAMES E. "Vision and Traffic Safety," *Sight-Saving Review,* Vol. 28, No. 3, 1958.

LEE, C. E. "Driver Eye Height and Related Highway Design Features," *Highway Research Board Proceedings,* Vol. 39, 1960, 46–60.

LEHMANN, KONSTANTIN. "Research into Causes of Road Accidents (Motorcycles and Automobiles)," *Australian Road Research,* Vol. 1, No. 4, Dec. 1962, 46–47.

LEIPPER, DALE F. *Fog Bibliography,* Scripps Institute of Oceanography, Fog Project Report No. 1, 1947.

LEVINE, HARRY. *Automobile Driving: The Not So Simple Act,* Fall River, Mass., 1966.

LEYGUE, F., P. DUFLOT, and F. HOFFMANN. "Investigation into the Influence on Accidents of the Age of the Driver, His Driving Experience, and the Age and Power of the Vehicle," *Highway Research Abstracts,* Vol. 36, No. 10, Oct. 1966, 3.

LIPPMAN, OTTO. "Eye Screening," *Archives of Ophthalmology,* Vol. 68, Nov. 1962, 692–706.

LISPER, HANS-OLAF, *et al.* "Effects of Prolonged Driving upon a Subsidiary Serial Reaction Time," Department of Psychology, University of Uppsala, Sweden, Report 52, May 1968.

LISTER, R. D., and R. N. KEMP. "Skid Prevention," *Automobile Engineer,* Vol. 48, No. 10, Oct. 1958, 382–391.

——, and BARBARA M. MELSOM. *Car Seat Belts: An Analysis of the Injuries Sustained by Car Occupants,* Road Research Laboratory, Department of Scientific and Industrial Research, Middlesex, England, 6–11.

LIT, ALFRED. "Depth-discrimination Thresholds for Targets with Equal Retinal Illuminance Oscillating in a Frontal Plane," *American Journal of Optometry and Archives of American Academy of Optometry,* Vol. 43, No. 5, May 1966, 283–298.

——, WILLIAM O. SWYER, and ANTHONY J. MORANDI. "Effect of Background Wavelengths on Stereoscopic Acuity at Scotopic and Photopic Illumination Levels," *American Journal of Optometry and Archives of American Academy of Optometry,* Vol. 45, No. 3, March 1968, 195–203.

LOGAN, H. L., and E. BERGER. "Measurement of Visual Information Cues," *Illuminating Engineering,* Vol. 55, 1960, 507–508.

LUCKIESH, M. "On 'Retiring' and 'Advancing' Colors," *American Journal of Psychology,* Vol. 29, 1918, 186–192.

——. "Blue Light Undesirable for Blackouts," *Illuminating Engineering,* Vol. 37, No. 2, Feb. 1942, 113–114.

——. "Visual Acuity and Visual Tasks," *Illuminating Engineering,* Vol. 39, No. 7, July 1944, 429.

——, and FRANK K. MOSS. *The Science of Seeing,* D. Van Nostrand Co., New York, 1937.

——, and ——. "Contrast Sensitivity as a Criterion of Visual Efficiency at Low Brightness Levels," *American Journal of Ophthalmology,* Vol. 22, 1939, 274.

——, and ——. "New Method of Subjective Refraction Involving Identical Technics in Static and in Dynamic Tests," *Archives of Ophthalmology,* Vol. 23, May 1940, 941–956.

——, and ——. "Characteristics of Sensitometric Refraction," *Archives of Ophthalmology,* Vol. 25, April 1941, 576–581.

——, and ——. "A New Method of Subjective Refraction at the Near-Point," *American Journal of Optometry and Archives of American Academy of Optometry,* Vol. 18, No. 6, June 1941, 249–257.

——, and ——. "Ability to See Low Contrasts at Night," *Journal of Aeronautical Sciences,* Vol. 9, No. 7, May 1942, 261.

——, and ——. "Comparison of a New Sensitometric Method with Usual Technics of Refraction," *Archives of Ophthalmology,* Vol. 30, Oct. 1943, 489–493.

——, and A. H. TAYLOR. "Visual Acuity at Low Brightness Levels," *American Journal of Ophthalmology,* Vol. 27, No. 1, Jan. 1944, 53–57.

————, and S. K. Guth. "Sensitometric Method of Refraction-Theory and Practice," *American Journal of Optometry and Archives of American Academy of Optometry*, No. 75, Sept. 1949.

Ludlam, William M. "Orthoptics Treatment of Strabismus," *American Journal of Optometry and Archives of American Academy of Optometry*, Vol. 38, 1961, 369–388.

Ludvigh, Elek. "Visual Acuity While One Is Viewing a Moving Object," *Archives of Ophthalmology*, Vol. 42, 1949, 14–22.

Ludvigh, E., and J. M. Miller. "Study of Visual Acuity During the Ocular Pursuit of Moving Test Objects," *Journal of the Optical Society of America*, Vol. 48, 1958, 799.

Lyle, W. M., and Henry W. Hofstetter. "Modification of the Bio-Photometer for Alterocular Fixation Control," *Highway Research Board Bulletin 336*, 1962, 33–36.

Manheimer, Dean I, Glen D. Mellinger, and Helen M. Crossley. "Follow-up Study of Seat Belt Usage," *Research Review*, Vol. 10, No. 1, March 1966, 2–13.

"Man-Made Highway Hazards That Kill," *Popular Science*, Vol. 186, No. 5, May 1965, 104–108 ff.

Marcus, Konrad H. "Periscopic Rear Vision in Automobiles," Society of Automotive Engineers, Mid-Year Meeting, Detroit, May 20–24, 1968.

Marsh, B. W. "Aging and Driving," *Traffic Engineering*, Nov. 1960.

Marsh, Charles R. "Highway Visibility in Fog," *Illuminating Engineering*, Vol. 52, 1957.

————. "Are Taillights Safe?" *Small World*, VW of America, Spring 1967, 20–22.

Masters, Dexter. "Our Chrome-Plated Caskets," *Washington Post Book Week*, Jan. 23, 1966, 1–10.

Mayer, Albert J., and Thomas F. Hoult. *Motor Vehicle Inspection*, Wayne State University Public Relations Office, 1963.

McColgin, F. H. "Movement Thresholds in Peripheral Vision," *Journal of the Optical Society of America*, Vol. 50, 1960, 774.

McFarland, Ross A. "Psychological Effects of Oxygen Deprivation on Human Behavior," *Archives of Psychology* (Columbia University), No. 145, 1932.

————. "Anoxia: Its Effects on the Body," *Science*, Vol. 98, July 1943, 18–19.

————. "Human Factors in Highway Transportation Safety," paper delivered before annual meeting of American Mutual Alliance, Chicago, Ill., Oct. 30, 1951; *Highway Research Board Bulletin 60*, Jan. 1952.

————. "Human Variables in the Design and Operation of Highway Transport Equipment," *Society of Automotive Engineers Preprint No. 717*, Jan. 1952.

————. "Human Factors in Highway Transport Safety," *Harvard Public Health Alumni Bulletin*, May 1952, 11–16.

————. "Human Factors in Highway Safety," *Best's Fire and Casualty News*, Oct. 1952, 37–38, and 132–140.

————. "Human Engineering: A New Approach to Driver Efficiency and Transport Safety," *Society of Automotive Engineers Transactions*, Vol. 62, 1954, 335–345.

————. "Psycho-Physiological Problems of Aging in Air Transport Pilots," *Journal of Aviation Medicine*, Vol. 25, June 1954, 210–220.

————. "Medical Aspects of Traffic Accidents: An Epidemiological Approach to the Control of Motor Vehicle Accidents," *Proceedings of the Montreal Conference*, H. Elliott, ed., Sun Life Assurance Company, 1955.

————. "Research in the Field of Accidental Trauma," *Military Medicine*, Vol. 116, No. 6, June 1955, 426–435.

————. "Human and Environmental Factors of Automobile Safety," *Society of Automotive Engineers Transactions*, Vol. 64, 1956, 625–654.

————. "Human Factors in Highway Transport Safety," *Society of Automotive Engineers Transactions*, Vol. 64, 1956, 730–750.

————. "Psychological Aspect of Aging," *Bulletin of the New York Academy of Medicine*, Vol. 32, No. 1, Jan. 1956, 14–32.

————. "Prevention of Accidents in Aviation Ground Operations," *Shell Aviation News*, June 1956, 14–17.

————. "Human Factors in Aircraft Safety," *Aviation Bulletin*, No. 160, July 1956.

———. "Human Limitations and Vehicle Design," *Ergonomics,* Vol. 1, No. 1, 1957, 5–20.

———. "Human Variables in Highway Safety," *International Road Safety and Traffic Review,* Vol. 5, No. 3, 1957, 15–20.

———. "Motorist Injuries and Motorist Safety: Human Engineering and Automobile Safety," *Clinical Orthopaedics,* No. 9, J. B. Lippincott Co., Philadelphia, Pa., 1957.

———. "Psychological and Psychiatric Aspects of Highway Safety," *Journal of the American Medical Association,* Vol. 168, Jan. 1957, 233–237.

———. "Role of Preventive Medicine in Highway Safety," *American Journal of Public Health,* Vol. 47, No. 3, March 1957, 288–296.

———. "Health and Safety in Transportation," *Public Health Reports,* Vol. 73, No. 7, Aug. 1958, 663–680.

———. "Current Research in Road Safety in the United States of America," *Practitioner,* Vol. 188, 1962, 457–466.

———. "Experimental Studies of Sensory Functions in Relation to Age," *Ergonomics,* Vol. 5, No. 1, 1962, 123–131.

———. "Epidemiology of Motor Vehicle Accidents," *Journal of the American Medical Association,* Vol. 180, April 1962, 189–300.

———. "Role of Human Engineering in Highway Safety," *Human Factors in Highway Safety,* Boston, Mass., 1963, 208–229.

———. "Critique of Accident Research," *Annals of the New York Academy of Sciences,* Vol. 107, No. 2, May 1963, 686–695.

———. "Experimental Evidence of the Relationship Between Aging and Oxygen Want: In Search of a Theory of Aging," *Ergonomics,* Vol. 6, No. 4, Oct. 1963.

———. "Human Factors Engineering," *American Society of Safety Engineers Journal,* Vol. 9, No. 2, Feb. 1964.

———, and A. L. BARACH. "Relationship Between Alcholic Intoxication and Anoxemia," *American Journal of Medical Sciences,* Vol. 192, No. 2, 1936, 186–198.

———, and W. H. FORBES. "Metabolism of Alcohol in Man at High Altitude," *Human Biology,* Vol. 8, No. 3, 1936, 387–398.

———, and ———. "Effects of Variations in the Concentration of Oxygen and of Glucose on Dark Adaptation," *Journal of General Physiology,* Vol. 24, No. 1, 1940, 69–98.

———, and J. N. EVANS. "Alterations in Dark Adaptation Under Reduced Oxygen Tensions," *American Journal of Physiology,* Vol. 127, No. 1, 1939, 37–50.

———, and M. H. HALPERIN. "Relation Between Foveal Visual Acuity and Illumination Under Reduced Oxygen Tension," *Journal of General Physiology,* Vol. 23, No. 5, 1940, 613–630.

———, J. N. EVANS, and M. H. HALPERIN. "Ophthalmic Aspects of Acute Oxygen Deficiency," *Archives of Ophthalmology,* Vol. 26, Nov. 1941, 886–913.

———, L. M. HURVICH, and M. H. HALPERIN. "Effect of Oxygen Deprivation on the Relation Between Stimulus Intensity and the Latency of Visual After-Images," *American Journal of Physiology,* Vol. 140, No. 3, Dec. 1943, 354–366.

———, et al. "Effects of Carbon Monoxide and Altitude on Visual Thresholds," *Journal of Aviation Medicine,* Vol. 15, No. 6, Dec. 1944, 381–394.

———, M. H. HALPERIN, and J. I. NIVEN. "Visual Thresholds as an Index of Physiological Imbalance During Anoxia," *American Journal of Physiology,* Vol. 142, No. 3, Oct. 1944, 328–349.

———, ———, and ———. "Visual Thresholds as an Index of the Modification of the Effects of Anoxia by Glucose," *American Journal of Physiology,* Vol. 144, No. 3, Aug. 1945, 378–388.

———, ———, and ———. "Visual Thresholds as an Index of Physiological Imbalance During Insulin Hypoglycemia," *American Journal of Physiology,* Vol. 145, No. 3, Jan. 1946, 299–313.

———, and A. L. MOSELEY. "Carbon Monoxide in Trucks and Buses, and Information from Other Areas of Research on Carbon Monoxide, Altitude, and Cigarette Smoking," *Health, Medical, and Drug Factors in Highway Safety,* Sept. 1954, 4.17–4.33.

————, A. L. MOSELEY, and M. B. FISHER. "Age and the Problems of Professional Truck Drivers in Highway Transportation," *Journal of Gerontology,* Vol. 9, No. 3, July 1954, 338–348.

————, and BRUCE FISHER. "Alterations in Dark Adaptation as a Function of Age," *Journal of Gerontology,* Vol. 10, No. 4, Oct. 1955, 424–428.

————, A. DAMON, and H. W. STOUDT. "Application of Human Body Size to Vehicular Design," *Special publication No. 142 of the Society of Automotive Engineers,* Nov. 1955.

————, ———— and ————. "Anthropometry in the Design of the Driver's Workspace," *American Journal of Physical Anthropology,* Vol. 16, No. 1, March 1958, 1–24.

————, R. C. MOORE, and A. B. WARREN. "Why Drivers Have Accidents," *Public Safety,* April 1956.

————, and R. C. MOORE. "Human Factors in Highway Safety: A Review and Evaluation," *New England Journal of Medicine,* Vol. 256, April 25, May 2, May 9, 1957, 792–799, 837–845, 890–897.

————, and RICHARD G. DOMEY. "Bio-Technical Aspects of Driver Safety and Comfort," *Society of Automotive Engineers Transactions,* Vol. 66, 1958, 630–648.

————, and ————. "Experimental Studies of Night Vision as a Function of Age and Changes in Illumination," *Highway Research Board Bulletin 191,* 1958, 17–32.

————, and ————. "Human Factors in the Design of Passenger Cars," *Highway Research Board Proceedings,* Vol. 39, 1960, 565–582.

————, ————, and A. BERTRAND WARREN. "Night Visibility: Dark Adaptation as a Function of Age and Tinted Windshield Glass," *Highway Research Board Bulletin 255,* 1960, 47–56.

————, A. BERTRAND WARREN, and C. KARIS. "Alterations in Critical Flicker Frequency as a Function of Age and Light: Dark Ratio," *Journal of Experimental Psychology,* Vol. 56, No. 6, Dec. 1958, 529–538.

————, and ROLAND C. MOORE. "Youth and the Automobile," *Values and Ideals of American Youth,* E. Ginzberg, ed., Columbia University Press, 1960.

————, and ————. "Accidents and Accident Prevention," *Annual Review of Medicine,* Los Angeles, Annual Reviews, Inc., 1962.

————, *et al.* "Dark Adaptation as a Function of Age I," *Journal of Gerontology,* Vol. 15, No. 2, April 1960, 149–154.

————, and HOWARD W. STOUDT. "Human Body Size and Passenger Vehicle Design," *Special Publication No. 142A of Society of Automotive Engineers,* 1960.

————, and ————. "Ergonomics in Transport," *Medicine in Transport: Rail, Road, and Sea,* E. G. Norman, ed., Butterworths, London, 1964.

————, G. SIDNEY TUNE, and ALAN T. WELFORD. "On the Driving of Automobiles by Older People," *Journal of Gerontology,* April 1964.

McKESSON, JON. "Autos Need Eight Big Changes to Make Them Visually Safe," *Indianapolis Star,* Jan. 23, 1966, 1.

McLAREN, DONALD S. "Nutritional Disease and the Eye," *Borden's Review of Nutritional Research,* Vol. 25, No. 1, Jan.–March 1964.

"Medical Aspects of Driver Limitation," *Journal of the American Medical Association,* Vol. 187, Feb. 1964, 376.

MELDRUM, J. F. "Automobile Driver Eye Position," *Highway Vehicle Safety,* Safety Committee of the SAE Passenger Car Activity, 848 pp.

Merck Index, PAUL G. STECHER, ed., Merck & Company, Rahway, N.J., 1968.

METCALF, R. A., and R. E. HORN. "Visual Recovery Times from High Intensity Flashes of Light," *American Journal of Optometry,* Vol. 36, 1960, 623–633.

MEYER, ROBERT L. "A Man Named Smith," *Traffic Safety,* Vol. 65, No. 11, Nov. 1965, 12–14 ff.

MICHAELS, RICHARD M. "Human Factors in Highway Safety," *Traffic Quarterly,* October 1961, 586–598.

MICHON, J. A. "The Problem of Perceptual Motor Load," *Studies in Perception,* Institute for Perception RVO-TNO, National Defense Research Organization TNO, Soesterberg, The Netherlands, 1966, 81–91.

MIDDLETON, W. E. K., and G. W. WYSZECKI. "Visual Thresholds in the Retinal Periphery for Red, Green, and White Signal Lights," *Journal of the Optical Society of America,* Vol. 51, 1960, 54–56.

MIDDLETON, W. E. *Vision Through the Atmosphere,* University of Toronto Press, Canada, 1952; Reprint, Oxford University Press, London, 1958.

MILLER, J. W. "Study of Visual Acuity During the Ocular Pursuit of Moving Test Objects, II," *Journal of the Optical Society of America,* Vol. 48, 1958, 803.

———, and E. LUDVIGH. "Effect of Relative Motion on Visual Acuity," *Survey of Ophthalmology,* Vol. 7, 1962, 83.

MILLER, H. GENE. "More About Small Cars," *United States Navy Medical News Letter,* Vol. 48, Oct. 1966, 23–24.

Minnesota Mining and Manufacturing Co. *This Could Save Your Life,* 3M Co., Reflective Products Division, St. Paul, Minn., 1964.

MIZOI, Y., S. HISHIDA, and Y. MAEBA. "Diagnosis of Alcohol Intoxication by the Optokinetic Test," *Quarterly Journal of Studies on Alcohol,* Part A, Vol. 30, No. 1, March 1969.

MOORE, GEORGE. "Three-colored Safety Taillights to be New Car Feature," *Indianapolis Star,* Feb. 16, 1966.

MOORE, R. L. "Forward Visibility from Vehicles," Department of Scientific and Industrial Research, Road Research Laboratory, England, October 1952 (mimeo.), 4.

———. "Rear Lights of Motor Vehicles and Pedal Cycles," *Road Research Technical Paper No. 25,* Her Majesty's Stationery Office, London, 1952.

———, A. CRAWFORD, and P. ODESCALCHI. "Driver Characteristics and Behavior Studies," *Highway Research Board Bulletin 25,* 1958, 104–120.

MOORE, R. L., and H. P. R. SMITH. "Visibility from the Driver's Seat: The Conspicuousness of Vehicles, Lights, and Signals," paper 6, *Ergonomics and Safety in Motor Car Design,* published by the Institution of Mechanical Engineers (1 Birdcage Walk, Westminster, London, SW1), Sept. 27, 1966.

———, and S. J. OLDER. "Pedestrians and Motor Vehicles Are Compatible in Today's World," *Traffic Engineering* (British), Sept. 1965.

MORTIMER, R. G. "Psychological Considerations in the Design of an Automobile Rear Lighting System," *Traffic Safety Research Review,* Vol. 12, No. 1, 1968, 13–16.

———. "Dynamic Evaluation of Automobile Rear Lighting Configurations," *Research,* No. 4, Highway Safety Research Institute, University of Michigan, March 1969.

———. "Dynamic Evaluation of Automobile Rear Lighting Configurations," *Highway Research Record 275,* 1969.

———, and P. L. OLSON. "Variables Influencing the Attention-Getting Quality of Automobile Front Turn Signals," *Traffic Safety Research Review,* Vol. 10, No. 3, 1966, 83–88.

MOSELEY, ALFRED L., *et al.* "Research on Fatal Highway Collisions," *Papers,* Harvard Medical School, Boston, 1961–62.

———, *et al.* "Research on Fatal Highway Collisions," *Papers,* Harvard Medical School, Boston, 1962–63.

"Motor Vehicle Accidents, 1967" *Accident Facts,* 1968, 40–45.

"Motorcycle Accidents—An Epidemic," *Highway Research Abstracts,* Vol. 36, No. 12, Dec. 1966, 94.

MOYNIHAN, DANIEL P. "An Opinion About Traffic Accident Statistics," *Highway Research Abstracts,* Vol. 36, No. 6, June 1966, 2.

MULLER, G. E. "Zur Theorie des Stabchenapparates und der Zapfenblindheit," Zeitschrift für Sinnesphysiologie, Vol. 54, No. 9, 1922–23, 102.

MULLIN, E. F. "The Part Visibility Could Play in Road Design," *Australian Road Research,* Vol. 2, No. 9, Sept. 1966, 15–43.

MUNKER, H. "Experimentelle Untersuchungen zur dynamischen Sehscharfe," Sonderabdruck aus, Bericht uber die 68, zusammenkunft der Deutschen Ophthalmologischen Gesellschaft in Heidelberg, 1967.

NADER, RALPH. *Unsafe at Any Speed: The Designed-in Dangers of the American Automobile,* Grossman Publishers, New York, 1965.

NADELL, M. C., and H. A. KNOLL. "Effect of Luminance, Target Configuration and

Lenses Upon the Refractive State of the Eye, Part I," *American Journal of Optometry and Archives of the American Academy of Optometry,* Vol. 23, 1956, 24–42.

NATHAN, JOHN, GEOFFREY H. HENRY and BARRY L. COLE. "Recognition of Colored Road Traffic Light Signals by Normal and Color-Vision-Defective Observers," *Journal of the Optical Society of America,* Vol. 54, No. 8, Aug. 1964, 1041–1045.

National Academy of Sciences. "Medical Guides Offered to Improve Design of 'Unsuitable Ambulances,'" *News Report* (2101 Constitution Ave., Washington, D. C.), Vol. 9, No. 1, Jan. 1969.

National Commission on Safety Education. *Minimum Standards for School Buses,* National Conference on School Transportation, Washington, D.C., 1964.

————. *Selection, Instruction and Supervision of School Bus Drivers,* Washington, D.C., 2nd ed., 1964.

National Safety Council. *Guide to Traffic Safety Literature,* Vol. 10, Chicago, 1955–1965.

————. *Accident Facts, 1965,* Chicago, 1966.

————. *Guidelines to Slow-moving Vehicle Emblem Legislation,* Chicago, 1966.

National Traffic Safety Act, *H.R. 12548,* House of Representatives of Eighty-ninth Congress, Second Session, Washington, D.C., 1966.

NELSON, THOMAS M. "Efficiency of Two Dimensional Traffic Markers in Referring Command," *Human Factors,* Aug. 1964, 359–364.

New York Department of Motor Vehicles. *Feasibility Study of New York State Safety Car Program,* Albany, New York, 1966.

New York Department of Transportation. *1952 Annual Report* (28-11 Bridge Plaza North, Long Island City, N. Y. 11101), 1952, 20–21.

"Night Vision Problems Studied at Michigan Traffic Center Seminar," *Traffic Safety,* Vol. 65, No. 8, Aug. 1965, 29.

O'CONNELL, JEFFREY, and ARTHUR MYERS. *Safety Last, An Indictment of the Auto Industry,* Random House, New York, 1966.

O'CONNOR, LIAM. "Wanted: Effective Traffic Signs," *Optometric Weekly,* June 5, 1958, 1076–1077.

"Ode to the Road," *Time,* Vol. 86, No. 11, Sept. 1965, 32–34.

OLENSKI, Z., and N. W. GOODDEN. *Clearness of View from Day-fighter Aircraft,* Farnborough (England) Royal Aircraft Establishment, Report No. Aero 1862, Oct. 1943.

"On-Off Sunglasses," *New York Herald Tribune,* Jan. 23, 1966.

Ontario Medical Association. *A Guide for Physicians in Determining Fitness to Drive a Motor Vehicle,* Ontario, Canada, March 1964.

OPPENHEIMER, JESS. "Orientation Apparatus for Human Subjects," *Optometric Weekly,* October 24, 1968, 23–31.

"Optometrist and Safe Driving," *Journal of the American Optometric Association,* Vol. 31, 1960, 467–469.

OSMUNDSEN, JOHN A. "Science: Through a Glass Darkly," *New York Times,* Dec. 5, 1965.

OTT, JOHN N. "Effects of Wavelengths of Light on Physiological Functions of Plants and Animals," *Illuminating Engineering,* Vol. 60, April 1965, 254–261.

————. "Some Observations on the Effect of Light on the Pigment Epithelial Cells of the Retina of a Rabbit's Eye," *Recent Progress in Photobiology,* E. J. Bowen, ed., Academic Press, New York, 1965, 395–396.

OTTANDER, CHRIS, and HANNES EISLER. *Hysteresis in the Continuum of Subjective Angular Velocity,* Psychological Laboratory, University of Uppsala, Sweden, Report 17, June 1964.

PAIN, RICHARD. "Brightness and Brightness Ratio as Factors in the Attention Value of Highway Signs," *Highway Research Record 275,* 1969.

PARKER, JAMES F., ROBERT R. GILBERT and RICHARD F. DILLON. *Effectiveness of Three Visual Cues in the Detection of Rate of Closure at Night,* Biotechnology, Inc., 3219 Columbia Pike, Arlington, Va., March 1964.

PATRICK, L. M., and R. P. DANIEL. "Comparison of Standard and Experimental Windshields," *Research Review,* Vol. 9, No. 4, Dec. 1965, 99.

PECKHAM, R. H. "Effect of Exposure to Sunlight on Night-Driving Visibility," *Highway Research Board Bulletin 56*, 1952, 17–24.

——, and W. M. HART. "Association Between Retinal Sensitivity and the Glare Problem," *Highway Research Board Bulletin 255*, 1960, 57–60.

PHILLIPS, A. J., and ALAN RUTSTEIN. "Amber Night Spectacles, a Further Study," *British Journal of Physiological Optics*, Vol. 24, No. 3, 1967, 161–205.

PIRENNE, M. H. "Spectral Luminous Efficiency of Radiation," *The Eye*, Hugh Davson, ed., Academic Press, New York, Vol. 2, 1962, 65–91; see p. 67.

PITTS, D. G. "Transmission of the Visible Spectrum Through the Ocular Media of the Bovine Eye," *American Journal of Optometry*, Vol. 36, 1959, 289–298.

PLATT, F. N. "Operation Analysis of Traffic Safety, IV, Proposed Fundamental Research on Driver Behavior," *Traffic Safety*, Vol. 4, No. 4, 1960, 4–7.

——. *Traffic Safety Research: A Unique Method of Measuring Road, Traffic, Vehicle and Driver Characteristics*, Ford Motor Co., Dearborn, Michigan, 1962.

Polk County (Iowa). 1959 Motor Vehicle Accident Study, Aug. 26, 1960.

Port of New York Authority. *Running Lights, Final Report*, Traffic Engineering Division (111 Eighth Ave. at 15th St., New York, N. Y. 10011), Oct. 1968.

POTTER, BARRIE. "Perception of Relative Movements of Illuminated Objects Along the Visual Axis," *British Journal of Physiological Optics*, Vol. 18, No. 2, April 1961, 117–124.

President's Committee for Traffic Safety. *Health, Medical Care and Transportation of the Injured (Driver Licensing and Alcohol and Drugs)*, report distributed by Division of Accident Prevention, Public Health Service, 1960.

——. *Highway Safety Action Program*, Washington, D.C., 1966.

PRINCE, J. H., H. R. BLACKWELL and J. G. OHMART. *Comparative Legibility of Highway and Advertising Signs Under Dynamic Conditions*, Ohio State University Institute for Research in Vision, Report on Project No. 886, 1963, 17.

PRITCHARD, B. S., and H. R. BLACKWELL. "Preliminary Studies of Visibility on the Highway in Fog," University of Michigan, Engineering Research Institute, Vision Research Laboratories, Final Report No. 2557-2-F, July 1957.

——, and ——. "Optical Properties of the Atmosphere and Highway Lighting in Fog," *Highway Research Board Bulletin 191*, National Academy of Sciences—National Research Council Publication 617, Washington, D.C., 1958, 7–16.

Proceedings of Joint Vehicular Signal System Committee Meeting, Columbus, Ohio, Aug. 18, 1965.

PROJECTOR, T. H., K. G. COOK and L. O. PETERSON. *Analytic Assessment of Motor Vehicle Rear Signal Systems*, Century Research Corp., Contract No. F-11-6602, National Highway Safety Bureau, U. S. Department of Transportation, Jan. 1969.

"Provision of Safety Features for All Motor Vehicles Used in Interstate Commerce," *Congressional Record, Senate*, Feb. 23, 1965.

RAINS, J. D. "Signal Luminance and Position Effect in Human Reaction Time," *Vision Research*, Vol. 3, 1963, 239.

READING, R. W., and HENRY W. HOFSTETTER. "Extrahoropteral Stereopsis in Vehicle Operator Orientation," *Highway Research News*, No. 17, Feb. 1965, 84.

REESE, JOHN H. "Legal Nature of a Driver's License," *Highway Research Abstracts*, Vol. 36, July 1966, 5.

"Reflectorization—A Modern Safety Boon," *Fleet Owner*, Vol. 58, No. 4, April 1963, 98–99.

REHLING, C. J. Drug Impaired Driver, *Highway Research Abstracts*, Vol. 37, No. 4, April 1967, 3.

REID and CHANON. "Studies in Fundamentals of Highway Lighting," *Illuminating Engineering*, Vol. 31, 1936.

——. "Determination of Visibility on Lighted Highways," *Illuminating Engineering*, Vol. 32, 1937.

——. "Evaluation of Street Lighting," *Illuminating Engineering*, Vol. 34, 1939.

——. "A Street Lighting Evaluator," *Illuminating Engineering*, Vol. 35, 1940.

REILLY, RAYMOND E., *et al. The Translation of Visual Information Into Vehicular*

Control Actions, Biotechnology, Inc. 3219 Columbia Pike, Arlington, Va., Report No. 65-2, Oct. 1965.

REINECKE, ROBERT D., and D. MILLER. *Strabismus, A Programmed Text,* Appleton-Century-Crofts, N. Y., 1966.

REX, CHARLES H. "Advancement in Roadway Lighting," *Highway Research Board Bulletin 255,* 1960, 158–189.

———. "Effectiveness Ratings for Roadway Lighting," *Illuminating Engineering,* July 1, 1963, 501–520.

———. *Light Distribution for the Motorist,* General Electric Company, Hendersonville, N. C., 1966.

———. "Visual Data on Roadway Lighting," *Highway Research Board Bulletin 336,* 1962, 61–75.

———, and J. S. FRANKLIN. "Visual Comfort Evaluations of Roadway Lighting," *Highway Research Board Bulletin 255,* 1960, 101–116.

———, and ———. "Relative Visual Comfort Evaluations of Roadway Lighting," *Illuminating Engineering,* Vol. 55, 1960, 161–174.

RICHARDS, OSCAR W. "Vision at Levels of Night Road Illumination, I (Reviews and Bibliography), *Highway Research Board Bulletin 56,* 1952, 36–55.

———. "Vision at Levels of Night Road Illumination, II," *Highway Research Board Bulletin 146,* 1957, 58–66.

———. "Vision at Levels of Night Road Illumination, III, Literature, 1956–57," *Highway Research Board Bulletin 191,* 1958, 57–61.

———. "Night Driving Seeing Problems," *American Journal of Optometry and Archives of the American Academy of Optometry,* Vol. 35, No. 11, Nov. 1958, 565–579.

———. "Night Driving Seeing Problems," *Traffic Safety Research Review,* Vol. 3, No. 2, 1959, 22–28.

———. "Vision at Levels of Night Road Illumination, IV, Literature, 1957–58," *Highway Research Board Bulletin 226,* 1959, 56–61.

———. "Vision at Levels of Night Road Illumination, V, Literature, 1959," *Highway Research Board Bulletin 255,* 1960, 190–195.

———. "Seeing for Night Driving," *Journal of the American Optometric Association,* Vol. 32, 1960, 211–214.

———. "What the Well-Dressed Deer Hunter Will Wear," *National Safety News,* Vol. 82, No. 5, 1960, 43–46, 104, 106, 108, 110, 112, 114, 124–127.

———. "Vision at Levels of Night Road Illumination, VI, Literature, 1960," *Highway Research Board RCS Circular 458,* 1961. 14pp.

———. "Vision at Levels of Night Road Illumination, VII, Literature, 1961," *Highway Research Board Bulletin 336,* 1962, 12–21.

———. "Vision at Levels of Night Road Illumination, VIII, Literature, 1962," *Highway Research Board Record 25,* 1963, 76–82.

———. "Do Yellow Glasses Impair Night Driving Vision?" *Optometric Weekly,* Feb. 27, 1964, 17–21.

———. "Vision at Levels of Night Road Illumination, IX, Literature, 1963," *Highway Research Board Record 70,* 1965, 41–47.

———. "Vision at Levels of Night Road Illumination, X, Literature, 1964," *Highway Research Board Record 70,* 1965, 67–73.

———. "Motorist Vision and the Driver's License," *Traffic Quarterly,* Jan. 1966, 16–17.

———. "Vision at Levels of Night Road Illumination, XII, Changes of Acuity and Contrast Sensitivity with Age." *American Journal of Optometry and Archives of the American Academy of Optometry,* Vol. 43, May 1966, 313–319.

———. "Visual Needs and Possibilities for Night Driving," *Optician,* Parts 1-12, Vols. 154–155, Nos. 3999–4006, 4008, 4011, 4012, 4015, Nov. 17, 24, 1967; Dec. 1, 8, 22, 29, 1967; Jan. 5, 12, 26, 1968; Feb. 16, 23, 1968; March 15, 1968.

———. "Night Myopia at Night Automobile Driving Luminances," *American Journal of Optometry and Archives of the American Academy of Optometry,* Vol. 44, No. 8, Aug. 1967, 517–523.

———. "Vision at Levels of Night Road Illumination, XI, Literature, 1965," *Highway Research Board Record 164,* 1967, 21–28.

———. "Vision at Levels of Night Road Illumination, XII, Literature, 1966," *Highway Research Board Record 179,* 1967, 61–67.

RILEY, H. "Driving in Dark Glasses," *Optician,* Vol. 140, 1960, 22.

RITTER, P. *Planning for Man and Motor,* (Hamilton and Thurstone quoted), Macmillan Company, New York, 1964, 58.

RIVERS, W. H. R. "Vision," in Schaefer's *Text-book of Physiology,* Vol. 2, London, 1900, 1091.

ROCKWELL, THOMAS H. "Visual Factors in Automobile Driving," *Proceedings, Symposium on Visibility in the Driving Task,* sponsored by Highway Research Board, Illuminating Engineering Research Institute, and Texas A & M University, May 13–15, 1968, 17–43.

———, and JOSEPH TREITERER. *Sensing and Communication Between Vehicles,* National Cooperative Highway Research Program Report 51, Highway Research Board, National Academy of Sciences–National Academy of Engineering, 1968.

ROPER, VAL J. "Aiming for Better Headlighting." Preprint copies available from SAE Headquarters, 485 Lexington Ave., New York 17, N. Y.

———. "Nighttime Seeing through Heat-Absorbing Windshields," *Highway Research Board Bulletin 68,* 1953, 16–17.

———. "Relation of Visual Acuity and Contrast Sensitivity Under Nighttime Driving Conditions," *Highway Research Board Bulletin 336,* 1962, 114.

———, and E. A. HOWARD. "Seeing with Motor Car Headlights," *Transactions of the Illuminating Engineering Society,* Vol. 33, No. 5, May 1938.

———, and K. D. SCOTT. "Silhouette Seeing with Motor Car Headlamps," paper presented before the annual convention of the Illuminating Engineering Society, San Francisco, Aug. 21–25, 1939.

———, and ———. "Seeing with Polarized Headlamps," *Illuminating Engineering,* Vol. 36, No. 12, Dec. 1941, 1205–1218.

———, and MEESE, G. E. "Seeing Against Headlamp Glare," *Illuminating Engineering,* Vol. 47, No. 3, March 1952.

———, and ———. "More Light on the Headlighting Problem," *Highway Research Board Bulletin 70,* 1964.

ROSS, H. L. "Recognition of Collision Course in Traffic Accidents," *National Safety Council Transactions,* Vol. 24.

ROTH, W. J., and F. DeROSE, JR. "Interchange Ramp Color Delineation and Marking Study," Michigan Department of Highways, Dec. 1964, for presentation at Highway Research Board annual meeting, Washington, D. C., Jan. 1965.

ROUSE, KENNETH A. *The Way To Go,* Chicago, Ill., Kemper Insurance Group.

ROWAN, NEILON J. "Tower Lighting Research," *Proceedings, Symposium on Visibility in the Driving Task,* sponsored by Highway Research Board, Illuminating Engineering Research Institute, and Texas A & M University, May 13–15, 1968, 124–129.

———, and NED E. WALTON. "Optimization of Roadway Lighting Systems," *Highway Research Record 216,* 1968, 34–47.

———, et al. *Impact Behavior of Sign Supports—II,* Texas Transportation Institute, College Station, Texas, 1965.

RUEDEMAN, A. D. "Foveal Coordination," *American Journal of Ophthalmology,* Vol. 36, 1953, 1220.

RUGABER, WALTER. "U. S. Plans Strict Safety in 1968 Autos," Louisville (Ky.) *Courier–Journal,* Feb. 17, 1966, 1.

RUMAR, KARE. *Visual Performance in Night Driving: A Summary of Some Research Results,* Department of Psychology, Universiy of Uppsala, Sweden, 1962.

———. "Night Driving Visibility," *Traffic Engineering and Control,* Feb. 1964, 611–613.

———. *Visible Distances in Night Driving with Misaligned Meeting Dipped Headlights,* Psychological Laboratory, University of Uppsala, Sweden, Report 28, Aug. 1965.

———. "Comparison of the Visibility and Readability between Conventional License Plates and License Plates with a Reflective Background," *International Police Chronicle,* No. 70, Jan-Feb. 1965, 21–44.

————. *Night Driving: Visibility of Pedestrians,* International Road Safety Congress reprint, 1966.

————. *Reflective Registration Plate,* paper delivered before Fifth World Meeting of International Road Federation, London, Sept. 1966.

RUSSELL, A. "Psychological Investigation of Glare in Road Traffic," *Highway Research Abstracts,* Vol. 28, No. 6, 1958, 2–3.

RUTTER, RICHARD. "Auto Industry Finds New Ways to Use Glass," *New York Times,* Jan. 3, 1966.

RYAN, JAMES J. "Safe Car," *Minnesota Medicine,* Vol. 43, No. 12, Dec. 1960, 869–870.

————, and JAMES R. TOBIAS. "Reduction in Crash Forces," *Proceedings of the Ninth Stapp Car Conference,* 1966, 413–419.

"Safety Experts Find Driver Behavior Prominent Cause of Accidents," *News Report,* Vol. 16, No. 4, April 1966, 5.

SAID, F. S., and ROBERT A. WEALE. "Variation with Age of the Spectral Transmissivity of the Living Human Crystalline Lens," *Gerontologia* (London), 1959, 213–231.

SAVIN, L. H., H. C. WESTON, and G. GRIME. "Discussion of the Visual Problems of Night Driving," *Proceedings of the Royal Society of Medicine,* Vol. 50, 1957, 173–184.

"Scanning the News: Drinking Drivers," *AMA News,* March 28, 1966.

SCHALLER, LYLE E. "How Free Are the Freeways?" *Highway Research Abstracts,* Vol. 36, No. 6, June 1966, 4.

SCHAPERO, MAX, DAVID CLINE and HENRY W. HOFSTETTER, eds., *Dictionary of Visual Science,* Chilton Book Co., Philadelphia, 1968.

SCHEIDT, EDWARD, D. J. MOFFIE and C. R. MILTON. *North Carolina Vision Program,* North Carolina Department of Motor Vehicles, 1954.

SCHMIDT, I. "Are Meaningful Night Vision Tests for Drivers Feasible?" *American Journal of Optometry,* Vol. 38, June 1961, 295–348.

————, and PAUL L. CONNOLLY. *Visual Considerations of Man, the Vehicle and the Highway,* Society of Automotive Engineers, New York, N. Y., 1966.

SCHOBER, HERBERT. "Unfersuchungen uber die Blendungsfrage, im besondersen uber die Blendung bei Gelblicht," Sonderdruck aus dem Tagungsbericht des IV. Internationalen Kolloquiums der Hockschule für Elektrotechnik Ilmenau, 1959, Vorstand des Instituts für medizinische Optik der Universitat Munchen.

————. "Optische und Optometristische Probleme bei der Bekampfung der Blendung bei Nacht und im Strabenverkehr (Optical and Optometrical Problems at Antiglare-fight and Night Traffic), Sonderdruck aus Internationaler, Augenoptiker-Kongreb, Kopenhagen, 1964.

————. "Role of Exact Eye Correction in Industrial Hygiene," *Sehanforderungen bei der Arbeit,* by Schmidtke and Schober, A. W. Gentner Verlag, Stuttgart, 1967, 96pp.

————. "Reduction of Disability and Discomfort Glare in Traffic," *Prevention of Highway Injury.* Proceedings of April 19–21 Symposium, Highway Safety Research Institute, University of Michigan, 1967, 99–112.

————, and H. MUNKER. "Blendschutzbrillen Gelbrillen," Sonderdruck, aus der Fachzeitschrift der Augenoptiker, Dusseldorf, Heft, 6/1968.

————, ———— and GRIMM. "Recognition of Moving Objects (Dynamic VA), "Klinische Monatsblätter für Augenheilkunde, 1967, 151, 399.

SCHOPPERT, DAVID W., and DAN W. HOYT. "Factors Influencing Safety at Highway-Rail Grade Crossings," National Cooperative Highway Research Program Report 50, Highway Research Board, National Academy of Sciences–National Academy of Engineering, 1968.

SCHRENK, L. S. "Street Lighting and Safety," *Illuminating Engineering,* Vol. 33, 1938.

SCHULTZ, HASKELL B. *A design for Safe Driving,* 3rd ed., Fort Wayne, Ind. 1963.

SCHUSTER, D. H. "Prediction of Current Accident Board for Youthful Drivers," *Research Review,* Vol. 10, No. 1, March 1966, 22–25.

SEARS, B. G. "Highways as Environmental Elements." Presented at 44th annual meeting of Highway Research Board, Jan. 1965.

"Seat Belts and Damages Collection," *Traffic Safety,* July 1967.

SEBURN, T. J. "Street Lighting—Traffic Accidents—Crime," *Illuminating Engineering,* Vol. 46, 1951.

SEEDORFF, H. H. "Effect of Alcohol on the Motor Fusion Reserves and Stereopsis as well as on the Tendency to Nystagmus," *Acta Ophthalmologica*, Vol. 34, 1956, 273–280.

SELZER, MELVIN L., and SUE WEISS. "Alcoholism and Traffic Fatalities: Study in Futility," *Highway Research Abstracts*, Vol. 36, No. 10, Oct. 1966, 4.

———, PAUL GIKAS and DONALD HUELKE, eds. *Prevention of Highway Injury*, University of Michigan, Highway Safety Research Institute, Ann Arbor, 1967.

SEPTON, RICHARD D. *Apparent Brightness Increases with Yellow Light*, Master's thesis, Indiana University, Aug. 1968.

SEVERY, DERWYN M. "Facial Injuries—Causes and Prevention," *Seventh Stapp Car Crash Conference Proceedings*, Charles C Thomas, Springfield, Ill., 1965.

———. "Survival by Design—Head Protection," *Seventh Stapp Car Crash Conference Proceedings*, Charles C Thomas, Springfield, Ill., 1965.

SHAW, LYNETTE. "Practical Use of Protective Personality Tests as Accident Predictors," *Traffic Safety Research Review*, Vol. 9, No. 2, June 1965, 34–72.

SHEEHE, G. H. "Importance of Driver Licensing Activities," *Optometric Weekly*, Vol. 51, 1960, 2566–2569.

SHERMAN, REUEL A. *Optometric Service in the Field of Automotive Driving*, Bausch and Lomb Optical Co., Rochester, N. Y., 1954.

SHERWOOD, STEPHEN L., ed. "Self-Induced Epilepsy," *Archives of Neurology*, Vol. 6, 1962, 49–65.

SHIPLEY, T. "Visual Efficiency in Monocular Driving," *Highway Research Board Bulletin 127*, 1955, 53–62.

SIEBECK, R. "Praktische Bedeutung der Raumsinnstorung durch Anisokorie," *Klinische Monatsblätter für Augenheilkunde*, Vol. 123, 1953, 86.

SIMMONS, A. E. "Instrument for Assessment of Visibility Under Highway Lighting Conditions," *Highway Research Board Bulletin 336*, 1962, 76–94.

SLOAN, L. L. "New Test Charts for the Measurement of Visual Acuity at Far and Near Distances," *American Journal of Ophthalmology*, Vol. 48, 1959, 807–813.

———, and S. M. NEWHALL. "Comparison of Cases of Atypical and Typical Achromatopsia," *American Journal of Ophthalmology*, Vol. 25, 1942, 945.

SMEED, R. J. "Some Factors Affecting Visibility from a Driver's Seat and Their Effect on Road Safety." *British Journal of Physiological Optics*, Vol. 10, No. 2, June 1953, 63–84.

———. "Proneness of Drivers to Road Accidents," *Nature*, Vol. 186, 1960, 273–275.

———. "Some Aspects of Pedestrian Safety," *Journal of Transport Economics* (London School of Economics and Political Science, Houghton St., Aldwych, London, WC 2), Vol. 2, No. 3, Sept. 1968, 255–279.

SMITH, K. U., *et al.* "Application of a Real-Time Computer System to the Clinical Treatment of Photosensitive Epilepsy," *Engineering in Medicine and Biology, Proceedings of the 19th Annual Conference, 1966*, Vol. 18, No. 4, 1966, 126.

"Smoke Dims Drivers' View," *Science News*, Vol. 90, Sept. 1966, 224.

SNELLER, ROBERT C. "Introducing Special Session on Highway Safety," *Journal of the American Optometric Association*, Vol. 32, 1960, 210.

———. "Vision and Its Correct Use in Safe Driving," *Optometric Weekly*, Vol. 51, 1960, 2551–2555.

———. *Vision and Driving*, American Optometric Association, St. Louis, Mo., 1962.

SNYDER, HARRY L., and CHARLES P. GREENING. *Effect of Direction and Velocity of Relative Motion Upon Dynamic Visual Acuity*, Washington, D.C., Department of Commerce, 1965.

Society of Automotive Engineers. *Lighting Equipment and Photometric Tests*, SAE, 485 Lexington Ave., New York, N. Y., May 1960.

———. *Design Aspects for Rear Vision in Motor Vehicles*, SAE, March 1964.

———. "Emblem for Identifying Slow-Moving Vehicles" (Corresponds to SAE J943) published by SAE, adopted by ASAE Dec. 1964.

———. *Proceedings of the Eighth Stapp Car Crash Conference*, Oct. 1964.

———. *Proceedings of the Ninth Stapp Car Crash Conference*, 1965.

———. *Proceedings of the Tenth Stapp Car Crash Conference*, Nov. 1966.

———. *Proceedings of the Eleventh Stapp Car Crash Conference*, Oct. 1967.

———. *Proceedings of the Twelfth Stapp Car Crash Conference*, 1968.

SOLOMON, DAVID. *Accident Involvements on Main Rural Highways Related to Speed and Characteristics of Drivers and Vehicles,* U. S. Department of Commerce, Bureau of Public Roads, Washington, D.C., 1963.

————. *Accidents on Main Rural Highways Related to Speed, Driver, and Vehicle,* U. S. Department of Commerce, Bureau of Public Roads, Washington, D.C., 1964.

SORSBY, A., *et al.* "Vision, Visual Acuity and Ocular Refraction of Young Men," *British Medical Journal,* Vol. 183, 1960, 1394–1398.

SPENCER, D. E., and S. C. PEEK. "Adaptation on Runway and Turnpike," *Illuminating Engineering,* Vol. 55, 1960, 371–384.

STALDER, H. E., and A. R. LAUER. "Effect of Pattern Distribution on Perception of Relative Motion in Low Levels of Illumination," *Highway Research Board Bulletin 56,* 1952, 25–35.

Stanford Research Institute. "Literature Search and Evaluation of the Physics of Fog," Report No. 1, Feb. 16, 1953.

STARKS, H. J. H. "Vehicle Design in Relation to Safety: Some Aspects of the Work of the Road Research Laboratory," *Medicine, Science, and the Law* (British), Oct. 1962, 469–481.

STEWART, CHARLES R. "Demonstration of the Effects of Alcohol on Vision," *Journal of the American Optometric Association,* Vol. 35, No. 4, 1964, 289–290.

STILES, W. S., and C. DUNBAR. "Evaluation of Glare from Motor Car Headlights," Technical Paper No. 16, Illumination Research Department of Scientific and Industrial Research, His Majesty's Stationery Office, England, 1935.

STONEX, K. A. "Review of Vehicle Dimensions and Performance Characteristics," *Highway Research Board Proceedings,* Vol. 39, 1960, 467–478.

————. "Roadside Design for Safety," *Traffic Safety Research Review,* Vol. 5, No. 4, 1961, 18–30.

————. "Vehicle Aspects of the Highway Safety Problem," *Traffic Safety Research Review,* Vol. 6, No. 2, 1962, 15–24.

————. "Relation of Cross-section Design and Highway Safety," *Traffic Safety Research Review,* Vol. 7, No. 4, 1963, 2–14.

STRAUB, A. L., and T. M. ALLEN. "Sign Brightness in Relation to Position, Distance, and Reflectorization, *Highway Research Board Bulletin 146,* 1957, 13–44.

STRICKLAND, J., and B. WARD. "Some Observations of the Pulfrich Type Distortions while Driving," in preparation.

STRUGHOLD, H. "Human Time Factor in Flight," *Journal of Aviation Medicine,* Vol. 20, 1949, 300; Vol. 22, 1951, 100.

————. "Intermittent Light," *German Aviation Medicine, World War II,* Vol. 2, Dept. AF, Washington, D.C., April 1950, 972.

————. "Human Time Factor in Flight II. Chains of Latencies in Vision," *Journal of Aviation Medicine,* Vol. 22, 1951, 100.

STUCKEY, W. E., and K. A. Harkness. *Pertinent Facts Regarding the Slow-Moving Vehicle Emblem,* Ohio State University.

"Studies, Trials, and Resolutions concerning the Visibility and Legibility of License Plates," *International Police Chronicle,* No. 70, Jan-Feb. 1965, 52–61.

SUTRO, P. J. "Windshield Visibility Clearance," *Traffic Safety Research Review,* Vol. 1, No. 1, 1957, 15–28.

SWEARINGEN, JOHN J. *Tolerances of the Human Face to Crash Impact,* Federal Aviation Agency, Oklahoma City, Okla., 1965.

TARAGIN, A., and B. M. RUDY. "Traffic Operation as Related to Highway Illumination and Delineation," *Highway Research Board Bulletin 255,* 1960, 1–29.

TAYLOR, A. H. "Vision at Low Brightness Levels, I," *Illuminating Engineering,* Vol. 38, No. 2, Feb. 1943, 89–98.

TAYLOR, STANFORD E. *Eye Movement Photography with the Reading Eye,* Educational Development Laboratories, Huntington, N. Y., 1960.

THOMAS, LLEWELLYN. "Movements of the Eye," *Scientific American,* Vol. 219, No. 2, Aug. 1968, 88–95.

THORNDIKE, R. L. "Human Factor in Accidents with Special Reference to Aircraft Accidents," Report to School of Aviation Medicine, U. S. Air Force, Feb. 1951 (reprinted Jan. 1964 by U.S. Department of Health, Education and Welfare), 140.

"To Cut Crash Toll, AMA Advises Auto-Design Changes, Stricter License Standards (excerpts)," *Journal of the American Medical Association,* Jan. 26, 1957, excerpts printed in *Safety Standards.*

Todosiev, E. P., and R. E. Fenton. "Velocity Thresholds in Car-Following." Presented at 43rd annual meeting of Highway Research Board, Jan. 1964.

Torf, Arthur S., and Lucien Duckstein. "Methodology for the Determination of Driver Perceptual Latency in Car Following," *Human Factors,* Oct. 1966, 441–447.

"Traffic Control and Roadway Elements: Their Relationship to Highway Safety," *Research Review,* Vol. 10, No. 4, Dec. 1966, 103.

Traffic Safety Act of 1966, *S. 3005,* Senate of the Eighty-ninth Congress, Second Session, Washington, D.C., 1966.

Travelers Insurance Company. *Deadly Reckoning: The Travelers 1961 Book of Street and Highway Accident Data,* Hartford, Conn., 1961.

——. *Cowboys and Engines: The Travelers 1962 Book of Street and Highway Accident Data,* Hartford, Conn., 1962.

——. *Rushin' Roulette: The Travelers 1963 Book of Street and Highway Accident Data,* Hartford, Conn., 1963.

——. *The Casualty Count: The Travelers 1964 Book of Street and Highway Accident Data,* Hartford, Conn., 1964.

——. *A Tragedy of Errors: The Travelers 1965 Book of Street and Highway Accident Data,* Hartford, Conn., 1965, 29.

——. *You Bet Your Life: The Travelers 1966 Book of Street and Highway Accident Data,* Hartford, Conn., 1966.

——. *Was It Sudden? The Travelers 1967 Book of Street and Highway Accident Data,* Hartford, Conn., 1967.

——. *Attitudes and Platitudes: The Travelers 1968 Book of Street and Highway Accident Data,* Hartford, Conn., 1968.

Turner, H. J. "Interaction Between Fixed Lighting and Vehicle Headlights," *Australian Road Research,* Vol. 2, No. 3, March 1965, 13,19.

Ungar, P. E., and J. Barnett. "Vision and the Driver," *Highway Research Abstracts,* Vol. 37, No. 4, April 1967, 4.

——, and ——. "Vision and the Driver," Aspects Techniques de la Sécurité Routière, *CIDITVA Bulletin,* Centre International de Documentation sur l'Inspection et la Technique des Vehicules Automobiles (14 rue du Gouvernment Provisoire, Brussels 1), No. 27, Drpy, 1966, 3.1–1.9.

"Uniformity Important in Lighting," *Traffic Safety,* March 1968, 25.

United Nations Conference on Road Traffic, Vienna, Oct. 7–Nov. 8, 1968, United Nations Publication, New York, 1969.

U. S. Department of Commerce. "Manual on Uniform Traffic Control Devices for Streets and Highways," Bureau of Public Roads, June, 1961.

——. *Standard Alphabets for Highway Signs,* Bureau of Public Roads, 1961.

U. S. Department of Health, Education, and Welfare. "Binocular Visual Acuity of Adults: United States—1960–1962," Public Health Service Publication No. 1000, Series 11, No. 3, 1964.

——. *Alcohol and Accidental Injury Conference Proceedings,* U. S. Government Printing Office, Washington, D.C., 1965.

——. *Accidents,* U. S. Government Printing Office, Washington, D.C., Dec. 1964–Jan. 1965.

U. S. Public Health Service. *Binocular Visual Acuity of Adults,* Publication No. 1000, Ser. 2, No. 3, Government Printing Office, Washington, D.C., 1964.

——. *Facts of Blindness,* Superintendent of Documents, Government Printing Office, Washington, D.C.

U. S. Department of Transportation. *Rail-Highway Grade-Crossing Accidents* for the year ended Dec. 31, 1967, Federal Railroad Administration, Bureau of Railroad Safety, 1968.

——. *Federal Motor Vehicle Safety Standards,* Federal Highway Administration, National Highway Safety Bureau, Aug. 6, 1968.

——. *National Traffic and Motor Vehicle Safety Act of 1966,* First Annual Report, U. S. Government Printing Office, Washington, D.C. 1968.

"Vehicle Safety-Check News," 1968 National Vehicle Safety-Check (2000 K Street, N. W. Washington, D.C., 20006), sponsored by Auto Industries Highway Safety Committee with cooperation of Association of State and Provincial Safety Coordinators, Dec. 1968.

"Visual Acuity and Driving," *Traffic Safety*, March 1968, 24.

"Visual Acuity of Young Men," *Optician*, Vol. 139, 1960, 512–513.

"Visual Communication Between Motor Drivers," *Optician*, Vol. 139, 1960.

"Vision and Traffic Safety," *Journal of the California Optometric Association*, Vol. 27, 1959, 302–303.

"Visual Capabilities of the Automobile Driver: Effects of Glare," *Visual Factors in Automobile Driving*, Stanley S. Ballard and Henry A. Knoll, eds., Highway Research Board of the National Academy of Sciences–National Academy of Engineering, Washington, D.C., 1958, 11.

"Visual Requirements for Vehicle Driving," *Visual Factors in Automobile Driving*, Stanley S. Ballard and Henry A. Knoll, eds., Highway Research Board of the National Academy of Sciences–National Academy of Engineering, Washington, D.C., 1958, 5.

VOEVODSKY, JOHN. "Inferences from Visual Perception and Reaction Time to Requisites for a Collision-Preventing Cyberlite Stop Lamp," *Proceedings of the National Academy of Sciences*, Vol. 57, No. 3, March 1967, 688–695.

Vos, J. J. "Some New Aspects of Color Stereoscopy," *Journal of the Optical Society of America*, Vol. 50, 1960, 785–790.

———. "Letters to the Editors: The Color Stereoscopic Effect," *Vision Research*, Vol. 6, 1966, 105–106.

———. "Antagonistic Effect in Colour Stereoscopy," *Ophthalmologica*, Vol. 145, 1963, 442–445.

———. "Physiologic-Optical Aspects of Participation in Traffic," *Perspectives in Ophthalmology*, Report of the 1967 Post-graduate Courses held under the auspices of the Netherlands Ophthalmological Society and the. Medical Faculty of Rotterdam, 223–229.

———, and J. BOOGAARD. "Contribution of the Cornea to Entoptic Scatter," *Journal of the Optical Society of America*, Vol. 53, No. 7, July 1963, 869–873.

———, and M. A. BOUMAN. "Disability Glare: Theory and Practice," *Proceedings of Commission Internationale de l'Eclairage*, Brussels, 1959, 298.

———, and ———. "Contribution of the Retina to Entoptic Scatter," *Journal of the Optical Society of America*, Vol. 54, No. 1, Jan. 1964, 95–100.

WALD, GEORGE. *Molecular and Fine Structures of the Retina: Recent Progress in Photo-biology*, Academic Press, New York, 133–144.

WALDRAM, J. M. "Visual Problems in Streets and Motorways," *Illuminating Engineering*, Vol. 57, 1962, 361–375.

WALKER, JAMES T. "Slanting Disc Effect: A Kinetic Visual Stereophenomenon," *Optometric Weekly*, Nov. 14, 1968.

WALLER, JULIAN. *Guide for the Identification, Evaluation and Regulation of Persons with Medical Handicaps to Driving*, American Association of Motor Vehicle Administrators, Washington, D.C., 1967.

WALLER, JULIUS A., "Alcohol and Traffic Accidents: Can the Gordian Knot be Broken?" *Traffic Research Review*, Vol. 10, No. 1, March 1966, 14–21.

WALRAVEN, P. L., and H. L. LEEBEEK. "Recognition of Color Code by Normals and Color Defectives at Several Illumination Levels: An Evaluation Study of the HRR Plates," *American Journal of Optometry*, Vol. 37, 1960, 82–92.

WALTON, W. G., and H. KAPLAN. "Motorists' Vision and the Aging Patient," *Journal of the American Optometric Association*, Vol. 32, 1960, 215–216.

WAYNE, E. "Alcohol and Road Traffic," Proceedings of the 3rd International Conference (London, 1962), B.M.A. House, London, 1963.

WEALE, ROBERT A. "Retinal Illumination and Age," *Transactions of the Illuminating Engineering Society* (London), Vol. 26, No. 2, 1961, 95–100.

———. *Aging Eye*, H. K. Lewis, London, 1963.

WEBER, DAVID. "Vehicle Lighting," *Fleet Owner*, Vol. 60, No. 7, July 1965, 86–93.

WESTHEIMER, G. "Eye Movement Responses to a Horizontally Moving Visual Stimulus," *Archives of Ophthalmology*, Vol. 52, 1954, 932.

WESTON, H. C., and L. H. SAVIN. "Discussion on the Visual Problems of Night Driving," *Proceedings of the Royal Society of Medicine*, Vol. 50, No. 3, 1957, 173–179.

WHITESIDE, T. C. D. *Heat Flash and Dazzle from Nuclear Weapons: The Principles of Aircrew Protection and Some Experimental Devices*, Ministry of Defense, Flying Personnel Research Committee, Farnborough, England, 1967.

WHITTEMORE, RUSSELL G. "Today's and Tomorrow's Automotive Glass," Society of Automotive Engineers Mid-Year Meeting, Chicago, May 17–21, 1965.

———, J. C. WIDMAN and J. D. RYAN. "Tomorrow's Automotive Glass—A Dynamic Element in Car Design," *S.A.E. Journal*, Vol. 73, No. 9, Sept. 1965, 50–52.

WILKE, D. J. K. "Investigation of Visual Acuity of Drivers," *British Medical Journal*, No. 5174, 1960, 722–723.

WILLETT, T. C. "Criminal on the Road: A Study of Serious Motoring Offenses and Those Who Commit Them," *Highway Research Abstracts*, Vol. 36, No. 3, March 1966.

WILLIAMS, ROGER J. *Nutrition in a Nutshell*, Doubleday & Company, Garden City, N.Y., 1962.

WOHL, MICHAEL G., and ROBERT S. GOODHART, eds. *Modern Nutrition in Health and Disease*, Lea & Febiger, Philadelphia, 1964.

WOLF, ERNEST. "Effects of Age on Peripheral Vision," *Highway Research Board Bulletin 336*, 1962, 26–32.

———. "Glare and Age," *Archives of Ophthalmology*, Vol. 64, 1960, 502–514.

———, and MICHAEL J. ZIGLER. *WADC Technical Report: Relationships of Glare and Target Perception*, U. S. Air Force, Wright-Patterson Air Force Base, Ohio, 1959.

———, ———, and H. B. COWEN-SOLOMONS. "Variability of Dark Adaptation," *Journal of the Optical Society of America*, Vol. 50, 1960, 961–965.

———, ROSS A. MCFARLAND and MICHAEL J. ZIGLER. "Influence of Tinted Windshield Glass on Five Visual Functions," *Highway Research Board Bulletin 255*, 1960, 30–46.

———, and BRENDA MCGOWAN. "Effect of Light-Time: Dark-Time Ratio and Luminance on Peripheral Sensitivity to Flicker," *Archives of Ophthalmology*, Vol. 69, Feb. 1963, 241–250.

WORTMAN, ROBERT H. "Headlight Glare Related to Lateral Separation," *Proceedings, Symposium on Visibility in the Driving Task*, sponsored by Highway Research Board, Illuminating Engineering Research Institute, and Texas A & M University, May 13–15, 1968, 130–144.

WRIGHT, H. L. "Atmospheric Opacity, A Study of Visibility Observations in the British Isles," *Quarterly Journal of the Royal Meteorological Society*, Vol. 65, 1939, 411–442.

WRIGHT, K. A., and W. R. BLEVIN. "Night-Time Luminance of White Roadlines," *Australian Road Research*, Vol. 2, June 1965, 3–11.

WRIGHT, W. D. "Subjective Brightness and Contrast in Relation to the Visual Task in Night Driving," in Erik Ingelstam, ed., *Lighting Problems in Highway Traffic*, Pergamon Press, London, 1963, Vol. 2, 81–93.

WULFECK, JOSEPH W., ALEXANDER WEISZ and MARGARET RABEN. *Vision in Military Aviation*, WADC Technical Report 58-399, ASTIA Document No. AD 207780.

———, *et al. Vision in Military Aviation*, WADC Technical Report 58-309, Wright Air Development Center, Wright-Patterson Air Force Base, Ohio, Nov. 1958, 170.

———, D. F. JOHANSSEN and P. L. MCBRIDE. "Studies on Dark Adaptation, III: Pre-Exposure Tolerances of the Human Fovea as Measured by Contrast Sensitivity," *Journal of the Optical Society of America*, Vol. 50, 1960, 556–558.

WYATT and LOZANCE, "Effect of Street Lighting in the Night Traffic Accident Rate." *Illuminating Engineering*, Vol. 50, 1955.

"Yellow Headlights," *Ophthalmic Optician*, April 2, 1966, 363.

ZOLI, M. T. "Bibliografia Sulla Miopia Notturna," *Atti Fond. Ronchi*, Vol. 14, 1959, 93–111.

Index

Merrill J. Allen, O.D., Ph.D.

DR. ALLEN, Professor of Optometry at Indiana University, has long been interested in the problems of vision as they concern motorists. With more than 100 articles published in professional magazines and journals to his credit, many of them on this subject, he is regarded as the outstanding authority.

A native of San Antonio, Texas, he now lives and works in Bloomington, Indiana.